We Lost Our Baby

We Lost Our Baby

One Couple's Story of Miscarriage and Its Aftermath

Siobhán O'Neill-White
and *David White*

The Liffey Press

Published by
The Liffey Press
Ashbrook House
10 Main Street
Raheny, Dublin 5, Ireland
www.theliffeypress.com

© 2007 Siobhán O'Neill-White and David White

A catalogue record of this book is
available from the British Library.

ISBN 978-1-905785-20-9

Printed in the Republic of Ireland by Colour Books Ltd.

Contents

For our baby.
Even though you did not quite
make it into this world, you will be
etched in our hearts forever.

Introduction

Siobhán

THE SECOND TIME AROUND is much easier. That is what I had been told by so many mothers. So when I became pregnant for the second time and it felt different from the first one, I did not worry about it too much. Unlike my first pregnancy, I was not constantly enveloped in a haze of nausea. I assumed that my body was more experienced this time around and, as such, I did not put too much stock into the old wives' tale that "morning sickness is the sign of a strong baby".

When I suffered a miscarriage, at twelve weeks and three days, I was completely shocked. I don't even like the word "miscarriage". It's so formal. It sounds like something you would hear in a courtroom: "a miscarriage of justice". It does not do justice to the heart-wrenching experience of losing a baby.

That's what happened to me: *I lost my baby*. The little life that was growing inside of me slipped away and left me empty, stunned and heart-broken.

I was in denial for quite a while after it happened. When I finally did come around and started looking for answers, I did not realise it would be so difficult to find them. I thought I would be able to go to my local bookstore and pick up several books about losing a baby. I was wrong. I searched and searched but all I found was one book. It was hidden away, out of sight (maybe because this is a subject we are sometimes afraid to tackle?) and I had to ask a sales assistant to help me find it.

Apparently somewhere between a quarter and a third of all pregnancies end up with the loss of the baby and all I could find was one book about it. To add to this, it was a very factual book. As much as facts and statistics are helpful, I wanted to read about how this tragedy had affected other people. I wanted to know if I was normal. Were my reactions and emotions normal? Was I feeling how other women felt when this happened to them?

I could not find any books that dealt with the emotional trauma. So I decided to write down my own personal experience in the hope that, some day, someone else who has lost a baby can pick it up and find some solace in the knowledge that their feelings and reactions are normal. (That's another word I don't like – *normal* – because I don't think there are any "normal" reactions to such a heart-wrenching loss).

Most importantly, this is a book about hope. My wish is that it inspires you, the reader, to be hopeful about, and look forward to, the future.

Dave

WHEN WE LOST OUR BABY it was definitely the most confusing time of my life. As a "Man" I felt that I was just supposed to get on with it, look after my wife and pass on messages from well-wishers. This was not a time to feel sorry for myself; this is something that affects the women, and aren't we lucky that we don't have to go through it?!

It seems to me that a lot of the books on pregnancy, birth, babies and parenthood are either written by doctors or mothers. The birth of our first baby and the loss of our second baby affected me profoundly and I wanted to co-write this book with Siobhán for any dads who have been unfortunate to experience the loss of a baby. It's heartbreaking for us too. We shed tears as well and we should not be afraid to talk about that, or to show our feelings about it. We have come a long way from the days when men were not "real men" if they cried. It's OK for us to feel the loss and, most importantly, to be able to talk about our loss. It was my baby too and I also have a right to grieve.

Chapter 1

How It All Began

Siobhán's recollections . . .

I HALF-EXPECTED IT TO HAPPEN to me on my first pregnancy and would run to the bathroom every so often to check that I was *not*, in fact, bleeding. Luckily for me I had a good pregnancy (except for all the morning sickness) and a good birth (except for all the pain!) on my first baby and so I *thought* I knew a thing or two when I became pregnant for the second time.

My second pregnancy was quite unexpected; in fact, I was shocked to discover I was pregnant again so soon. It wasn't exactly planned.

My son was seven months old and my husband's Christmas party was coming up. I was starting to get the hang of this parenting business and my feelings of panic when leaving the baby at all had started to dwindle. That tends to happen when they start teething! Between sleepless nights and all the work that goes with a very active seven-month old, every so often we needed a break. We needed some time alone as a couple, so every now and then the grandparents would babysit. It was nice. The panic I felt as a new mammy was wearing off and I was getting a little bit of a social life back. I was feeling kind of like my old self again.

When my husband asked me if I wanted to go to his work Christmas party, adding that his parents had offered to take the baby overnight so that we could stay out late and sleep in the next day, I was very happy to say "yes". Having a night out to-gether was a rare treat and I was really looking forward to it.

We got the baby ready and my husband left him over with the grandparents while I spent ages get-ting ready. I did not get out much anymore, so I was making the most of it. We went along, had a lovely dinner and a few glasses of wine. We called and checked on the baby and he was sleeping fine, so my husband suggested we go to a nightclub. I love dancing but I suggested we go home. He was surprised and a little bit disappointed but when I told what I had in mind for him, he was pulling his coat on with record speed to run out and hail a taxi! (We had not been getting much "alone time" since the little nipper had come along, so the chance of an uninterrupted kiss and cuddle was far more appeal-ing than a nightclub).

We got home, cracked open a bottle of wine, put on some soft music and lit the fire. As we were getting down to the good stuff, we realised we had no contraception. You know the way it is (I should get a slap on the wrist for saying this); we had been sipping on wine for a while, the fire was warm and the little man was away for the night. It was tempting, to say the least. Add to that temptation the fact that it was a windy and rainy December night outside and the nearest chemist or shop was well past closing time so, even if we had tried, we may not have been able to find condoms; plus we were getting caught up in the heat of the moment and we did want to interrupt all that to sort out contraception. (I know, I know, we were very irresponsible . . .) Anyway, I calculated my dates and reckoned we were safe, so we threw caution to the wind and had a very pleasant night.

Two weeks later it was Christmas. I felt a little bit tired. I was a tad short-tempered as well. I just thought I was run-down from all the Christmas preparations. I was so tired on Christmas Day that I did not even have wine with my dinner and, soon after dessert, I was curled up on the sofa in my pyjamas. I thought my exhaustion was from a lack of sleep and the constant running around after a very energetic and imaginative seven-month-old.

It never dawned on me that I could be pregnant; I thought I was simply worn out from how busy I had been. Instead of thinking about my symptoms and putting two and two together, I put my feelings of tiredness down to the baby teething and the fact we had cooked for eight people on Christmas Day.

We had booked a winter holiday for the three of us. My husband and I had decided it would be our Christmas present to each other that year and we were really excited at the prospect of getting some sun, while it was freezing cold here. A few days into the New Year, we headed off to the Canaries for some sun and relaxation. I still felt a bit tired; I was expecting my period to arrive at any minute and I usually get a bit tired before it arrives. I never suspected for a minute that I might be pregnant. After all, we had only been together without contraception that one time, so I thought we were safe.

On our first night away we had dinner and ordered some wine. I was not really up to much and the smell of the wine did not appeal to me. Looking back now I should have realised what was going on but I was so preoccupied with my son that I thought all my feelings of tiredness were due to sleepless nights and all the travelling we had done that day. We had a pretty early night as we were all exhausted from the long day; also, we wanted to get up early the next morning, as we were planning to head off and explore the island in our hired car.

The next morning we hopped into the car and as we were heading up the main road out of the town, we came across a shopping complex. I must admit, I am something of a shopaholic, so I wanted to go in.

My husband reluctantly agreed, so we parked the car. Just as we walked in the front doors of the complex, I stopped and gagged. I was repulsed by the smell of fish. I could not even see a fish bar, so I did not know where the smell was coming from but I could not stand it. I had to run out of the centre to get some fresh air in a bid not to throw up. My husband, running after me, joked that I must be "up the duff". (He never was very eloquent!) I started putting two and two together. I did not like the smell or taste of wine. I was feeling very tired. I had been a bit ratty over the previous weeks. I could smell a fish counter at the back of a supermarket – from practically outside the supermarket. All signs indicated I was pregnant. Not quite believing I could be, I decided I had better get a test and find out for sure.

I went into a chemist and asked for a pregnancy test. I soon realised no-one could understand me, so I went off around the shop by myself, trying to find a test. After an unsuccessful search of the shop, I enlisted the help of the staff again. *Baby*, I gestured as I rubbed my tummy. They eventually figured out what I was saying and went into the back, into the stockroom, to retrieve a test for me. (It's a lot different from Ireland, where you can buy pregnancy tests at the front of the shop, well displayed). It was not like that in Lanzarote. They were very secretive about it. The tests were not on display anywhere in the shop. They were also very discreet; instead of handing it to me over the counter in full view of everyone, they had the test fully concealed and wrapped up in a brown paper bag, well out of sight, before they even let me pay for it!

We went back to the hotel, safely away from the fish bar, and I went into the bathroom to do the business. We waited in our room, on the bed, as our eight-month-old, who had just learned to walk around the furniture, was smiling and gurgling at us. I went back in. There were two pink circles waiting for me. The test was front to back in Spanish but I assumed that it is universally accepted that two blue lines, or two pink circles, mean "*si*", there is a baby. We celebrated, albeit a little apprehensively, as we watched our little boy walking, crawling and stumbling around the room. I'm sure we were both thinking the same thing: "How are we going to manage two, when we already have our hands full with this one?"

Still, we had always wanted more children and this way, they would be close together in age and they would be great pals. After the shock started to wear off, we talked about it and agreed that it was good news, even if was a little unexpected! I started calculating dates and I realised that our baby's due date would be September 11th. Everyone remembers the awful events of that date in 2001, but we decided not to take it as an omen. Our son, Mitchell, had been born ten days early so we hoped this little bundle of joy would be just as accommodating and come before his or her due date too.

We were lucky with the lovely hotel and warm weather, so we made the most of our time away by enjoying a relaxing and leisurely week. We did lots of sleeping and swimming and generally had a relaxing time. We were coming around to the idea of there being four of us soon. I was fast learning that, when it comes to babies, the word "planning" usually does not apply!

We went home rejuvenated and happy. Because I had already been through a good pregnancy first time around and was lucky enough to have a healthy baby, I did not think twice about telling my mother the good news when I was only six weeks' pregnant. I assumed everything would go fine because I had been through it all before and did not wait for the twelve-week "safety net" to pass before sharing my good news. When I said "Mam, you'll never guess what . . .", the expression on her face showed she was not expecting that kind of news at all. She was quite shocked but I assured her (I think I was reassuring myself too) that we were happy about and I asked that she be happy for us too.

Once she saw we were genuinely happy, she was great about it. She knew first-hand how hard it would be to have two babies close in age because my sister and I were born just twenty months apart but she reassured me (or maybe she was trying to comfort me!) that I would be fine. She told me how she had coped just fine with us two and she was sure I would manage too. She did admit that she found it a little bit hard when we were both small babies but that once we were toddlers, my sister and I occupied each other most of the time, by playing together. In the long run, she assured me that she was glad we had been so close in age because we were such good friends as a result. I knew she was deliberately avoiding telling me how hard it would be but I appreciated it at that time because truth be told, I was rather overwhelmed at the thought of having two babies with only sixteen months between them.

So the cat was out of the bag. My secret was not a secret for long. I did not worry that I had told her so soon because I assumed all would be fine. There was a lesson to be learned there as well (even though I did not know it at that point). You should never assume anything when it comes to pregnancy and babies. I know that now. I wish I had not been so quick to talk about it. I would have told my family but I would not have told friends and acquaintances so quickly. It's only later, when the baby is gone and you run into someone you know who has not heard that you lost your baby and who asks how the pregnancy is going, that you wish you could turn back time and keep your mouth shut. Even worse is when you run into someone you have not seen for a while. You know as they are talking to you at first they are staring at your tummy, looking for a growing bump and confused as to why you are not "showing". Sadly there is no bump any more and you have to explain and try to save yourself from tears and them from awful embarrassment – that's an awkward moment for everyone involved. I guess that's why our mothers and grandmothers kept tight-lipped until they had passed the three-month barrier.

I went to see my doctor when I was eight weeks pregnant and she confirmed my good news. I told her I was not experiencing any sickness or discomfort. I explained to her that I had suffered very badly from morning sickness on my first pregnancy and that I was a bit worried that I was not feeling any of that this time around. She told me not to worry about it. She assured me that all pregnancies are different and that what happened for me first time around, might not happen this time. So I went off home, feeling chuffed with myself that I was off the hook with the awful "morning, noon and night sickness", as I used to call it.

I called the hospital the next day and booked in for my first appointment. I was due to go there at fourteen weeks. I was starting to get excited about the pregnancy, especially since I had booked my scan appointment and would soon be able to see my little baby bouncing around inside me. All was going well. I felt OK and I was coming around to the idea of managing with two babies less than eighteen months of age!

Dave's recollections . . .

I WAS 30 WHEN MY SON WAS BORN. Up until then I could not remember crying, but his arrival certainly opened up something inside of me. Shortly after his birth, I was driving from the hospital to meet my parents and brother for the traditional celebratory drinks. As I was driving along, thinking about his little face and my beautiful wife and the over-whelming and amazing experience we had just been through, something weird happened. From nowhere I started to gush crying. It took me over completely and I had to stop the car for a few min-utes to calm myself. It was incredible. It was so powerful that I could not stop it for what seemed like the longest time. Finally, I got myself together and drove off to meet my family in our local.

As I entered the pub and proceeded to walk to-wards their table, it happened again. The tears were flying out of my eyes and I was unable to stop them. I'm sure it was as much of a shock to my par-ents and brother as it was to me, especially as I did not have as much as one drop of alcohol inside me, to account for my outburst. When the tears ceased and I finally got myself sorted, for the second time that day, I assured them that everything was fine and that I was just feeling very emotional from the birth and also tired from a lack of sleep.

This emotional release, which had never hap-pened to me before that day, was something that would surface again in a matter of months, but for totally different reasons . . .

When I found out that Siobhán was pregnant for the second time, I was delighted but a bit surprised because it was not planned. On this pregnancy, the first few months were very strange. I remembered *vividly* what a pregnant wife was like first time around. Loving, caring, affectionate – these were words that did not apply. Crazy, obsessive and deluded were closer to the mark; I still have the war wounds to show for it. However, this time was different. It was much more subdued and less frantic and emotional. In other words, I was not afraid of what mood she would be in when I got home from work. She was not throwing things or crying at the drop of a hat on this pregnancy. I remember reasoning that, because Siobhán had already carried a baby, her body and mind were used to this, so maybe that explained why she seemed more mellow. Also, the fact that we had such a young baby boy at home to keep her occupied kept her mind on other things. I thought it was just going to be easier second time around; how wrong I was to think like that.

Chapter 2

When It All Went Wrong

Siobhán's recollections . . .

Sunday Afternoon, February 23rd

MY HUSBAND'S PARENTS HAD AGREED to come over and watch the baby for an afternoon, so we could go to the cinema. We could not exactly go clubbing considering my condition (well, I suppose we could have but I suspect it would not have been a lot of fun, with me sipping on water), so the cinema was our new favourite pastime. We would head off to see a movie whenever we wanted a couple of hours out of the house. We had booked tickets for a comedy and I was looking forward to going.

Just before we were about to leave, I ran upstairs to the bathroom. One side effect of pregnancy I never enjoyed was the constant need to pee. I would automatically go to the bathroom whenever I was leaving the house, even if I didn't feel the need. I went in, peed the customary three drops and when I stood up I noticed a speck of blood on the toilet paper. It was just a tiny spot that I could easily have missed, but I didn't. My eyes were fixed on it as my heart sank. I knew at that exact moment that my baby was lost. That may sound like a very pessimistic thing to say; I know some women have bleeding in their pregnancies and the babies turn out fine but deep in my heart I knew that my baby was slipping away. I can't explain how and I did not want to believe it but somehow I just knew.

I screamed for my husband to come up and when he did, I showed him the little spot of blood. He was very calm and suggested that we ring one of the midwives in the hospital to ask if this was something to worry about. We called them and they assured us that it can happen in pregnancy and that quite often, it is nothing to worry about. They said I should carry on as normal and if it got any worse, I should go to see my GP.

I started to think quite differently about my pregnancy after I saw that speck of blood. I began to feel bad for not cherishing being pregnant, more than I had been, up to that point. So what if I would have two little nippers under the age of eighteen months? Suddenly that seemed irrelevant. All I wanted now was for my baby to be safe and healthy. *My baby*. I had not thought about my baby as much as I had thought about the actual pregnancy or what it would be like to have two small babies. I had been dwelling on the wrong things and the guilt of that was almost crippling. I had been focusing on things like how I would cope in the last few months, when I would be running after a fifteen-month-old and carrying around a big bump at the same time. However, once I saw the blood and felt the fear of what "could" or "might" happen, I vowed that I would definitely focus on my baby and my pregnancy all the more from that moment. If it was a lesson I was supposed to learn, then I had learned it. I would not take my baby or being pregnant for granted, as I had been doing. I was fast learning that life is very precious and extremely fragile and should *never* be taken for granted. I swore all these things to myself, in my head, as I hoped against hope that somehow it would all be OK.

My husband suggested that we go to the cinema as planned, to keep us distracted, and so off we went. We saw the movie (I don't remember too much but it did distract me at times), had something to eat and walked around for a while. I wanted to believe that everything would be fine but I had a niggling feeling that the worst was ahead of us. We went home and I was constantly running to the bathroom, checking for more blood. There was very little that day, but the few spots that did come caused me more worry than I had ever experienced in my life.

Monday Morning, February 24th

The next morning, as I got out of bed with trepida-
tion, I just knew it was worse. I could feel the blood
before I got to the bathroom. There was not a great
deal of it but it was enough to make me get to my
doctor's surgery for the first early morning appointment. The doctor we saw said we should try
not to worry (how on earth is that possible?) but to
ease our minds he called the hospital and asked
them to slot us in for a scan that afternoon.

We felt a bit relieved; surely the scan would
show that the baby was growing "normally"? I hate
to use that word but that's what we wanted them to
tell us. We wanted to hear that our baby was within
the "normal" size range for a twelve-week-old foetus. We wanted to see and hear the heart beating on
the scan. We wanted to see our baby bouncing
around on the monitor. We wanted reassurance.
We wanted some sort of *normality* to stop all this
worrying. It was driving me mad.

We went to the hospital that afternoon. It was
not the hospital where Mitchell was born. We had
experienced a few problems during his birth and
we thought we could do better second time around,
so we chose a different hospital. I suppose there
was a lesson to be learned there as well; the saying
"better the devil you know" springs to mind. At the
hospital where Mitchell was born there had been
problems with overcrowding and they were short-
staffed too. My birth experience had not been at all

how I had imagined it to be and I felt disappointed afterwards. I vowed to have a better experience second time around. I wanted to go somewhere where the staff would listen to me and where there would not be such a problem with overcrowding and staff shortages. We decided to try a hospital on the other side of the city that had been recommended to us.

I was stunned to discover it to be so much worse than where we had our son. When I gave birth the first time, I was not very happy with the overall experience but in hindsight I guess a lot of the aspects which I was disappointed with were out of the control of the staff. I have to say that the staff there were very friendly. Unfortunately I was about to find out the hard way that having helpful and friendly staff around you counts for a lot! They can make *all* the difference.

I could not have imagined there could be somewhere with fewer staff and less time for expectant mothers, but that's how it was. This other hospital was much, much worse. It was bare and cold and the staff were almost nowhere to be seen. We had to wait a long time and the staff did not seem too bothered about leaving us there for hours. When we eventually did meet the nurses and doctors who would be looking after us, they were not very pleasant or understanding and they did not go out of their way to reassure us either. Even if the situation had been totally hopeless, it could not have done any harm if they had been more sensitive and reassuring. A little pat on the shoulder or a smile would have gone a long way. It would have meant a lot to us at that time, when we were waiting to hear the fate of the little baby growing inside me. I'll never forgive or forget their easy-going approach to our gravely serious situation.

We waited for what seemed like a lifetime and eventually a nurse called me in. She took a urine sample from me and checked for the HCG pregnancy hormone. It came up positive, which was a good sign. It meant I was definitely still pregnant and that I was still producing that hormone. The signs were good. We had some hope.

We went back outside and waited for the doctor. After a long while, he arrived. First he asked me a few questions and then he asked me to lie on the table, so he could examine me and do an ultrasound scan. He started the scan but had difficulty finding the baby's heartbeat. He asked about my dates again and asked if they could be wrong.

I was pretty sure I had my dates right but, in the hope of finding out that the baby was small because I had mixed up my dates, I told him that I could have been wrong about them. Instead of what looked like a twelve-week-old foetus, he said our baby looked to be about six weeks old. He could not find a heartbeat. It was the tensest moment of my life. As he told me to relax so he could examine me, I could feel every muscle in my body tensing up. I knew I had to be strong so I tried my very best to relax as I lay there, panicking about whether or not my baby had any heartbeat. I knew our baby should have had a very strong, very visible heartbeat at twelve weeks but there and then, it seemed there was no heartbeat to be found.

He asked for my permission to do an internal ultrasound scan. These scans can be more accurate as they can get closer to the baby this way. They are uncomfortable for the mother, to say the least, but I agreed immediately because I was willing to go through anything at that stage to hear my baby's heartbeat. He began the scan and looked carefully for a heartbeat. He eventually found one, but it was weak. He said that we either had a six-week-old embryo, which would explain the weak heartbeat and that this would be nothing to worry about, or else we had a twelve-week-old foetus that was not forming properly – and this would be something to worry about.

We went home praying that we had our dates wrong. I knew in my heart that we didn't – but still I hoped. I was willing to fool myself for the smallest chance, just the slightest possibility, that I had them wrong and that the baby was only six weeks old. I was willing to trick myself into thinking that the baby was just not developed enough yet for a strong heartbeat to be present. It was a strange drive home that Monday afternoon but we tried to be positive – for each other and for our little baby, who was clinging on to life.

The doctor had arranged for us to come back on the Thursday for another scan to see how the baby was progressing. However, he said we could come back before then if the bleeding got any worse. We felt a bit more optimistic as we got home. The bleeding had not stopped but it had not got any worse either and so, I felt a glimmer of hope. I was very aware that Dave was full of hope and optimism and did not want to burst his bubble with my thoughts of doom and gloom, so I tried my best to be optimistic too. I tried to see the hope he was seeing and so we clung on to the smallest chance that things would work out alright.

Tuesday Morning, February 25th

The next morning the bleeding got worse. I was so worried. We went straight back to the hospital. We waited for the doctor to come and when he did, he suggested that the bleeding was indicative of a possible miscarriage. He looked at us and he actually said, "it probably just has not happened yet". Those were the cruellest words I have ever heard. I'm sure he did not mean to upset us but he spoke to us like he was talking about something of no importance. He seemed to be talking about a thing, not our little baby, who was, at that point, struggling to stay alive. This doctor, who was perhaps overworked, in one of our overcrowded hospitals, was more insensitive than anyone I have ever met in my life. He was so matter-of-fact about telling us our baby was probably going to die. He did not even blink as he said it.

I was beyond shocked at his cavalier approach to giving us this news. I would like to think he did not mean to be so hurtful because I always try to see the good in people but I struggled to see it in him. I generally think that people do not mean to be deliberately hurtful without cause. If someone is hurtful or rude to me I often think that I am just around them on a bad day; I do my best not to take it personally. But how could I not take his attitude personally? He was talking about my baby and he did not seem to care one little bit. I try to understand his behaviour by thinking that he has a very hard job, where he is possibly under-appreciated and maybe underpaid – but even when I put his attitude down to whatever possible frustrations he may have in his job, I cannot excuse the lack of humanity he expressed when he gave us that news.

I could feel the tears forming in my eyes as soon he uttered those words. I could feel the rage building up inside me over the way he referred to my baby. My baby, who was still inside me. My baby, who was a part of me. In my mind, he or she was already a part of our family. I had hopes and dreams that included this baby. I had names picked out. I had visions of Christmas with two babies. All of those hopes and dreams were crushed with one cold sentence from a doctor who just did not have the time or insight to be sensitive to our over-whelming sadness at what he was telling us.

My husband is not a violent man at all but when that doctor uttered those words, I could see a look of rage flash across his face. I looked at him and calmed him down with a scornful look that said, "Please don't punch him; he's not being insensitive on purpose." It would not have helped if Dave had punched him. It would not have helped if I had shouted or screamed at him. No matter what we said or did, he would not have given us any differ-ent news at that point. Nothing could stop what was happening but we could have been told in a more humane way – it would not have been as bad then.

I still think about that doctor now. I wonder how many women have had to hear similar sad news from such an uncaring person. I hope he has learned to be a bit more empathic. I do understand that doctors are very busy but I don't accept that there is *ever* a time for them to be complacent. This is even more important when it comes to parents and their children or babies – especially if there is a chance that the baby in question is not going to make it into this world. There is a time for doctors to be doctors but there is also a time for doctors to be human and that was one of those times. I'll never forget that doctor as long as I live. I know it was all in a day's work for him but it was some-thing that would affect the rest of our lives and a little compassion would have gone a long way.

We left the hospital shredded and devoid of hope. Not only were we facing the prospect of losing our baby but the doctor had not been explanatory or understanding about it. I wanted to know why my baby was not growing properly. I wanted to know if there was anything that we could do. I needed to speak to a doctor who could explain things to me. We decided to go straight over to the hospital where we had our first baby. We called them and asked if we could come in. As much as it was very busy, the doctors, midwives and nurses (even though they were seriously overworked) were understanding and empathic. That was exactly what we needed.

They might as well have rolled out the red carpet for us – that was how it felt. They were great. They brought us in and talked to us and explained things to us and told us that all hope was not lost. Far from it, in fact; and to give us even more hope, they booked us in for a special early pregnancy scan the very next morning. We were so optimistic when we left the hospital that Tuesday afternoon. We were looking forward to the scan the following morning. They had spent time explaining things to us. They had told us to be calm and positive because there was still a good chance that everything would be OK. The scan would tell us what we needed to know the next day and until then, they advised us to go home and relax as much as possible.

Even if they knew it was all going to end in disaster, in my opinion, they did the right thing by giving us some hope. Even though I still had feelings of dread that the worst was yet to come, I did feel a bit better and even momentarily gave myself permission to hope it might all work out. The next few hours were a happy few hours and I am so grateful for that. Either way, if our baby was not going to make it into this world, there was a world of pain waiting for us; so for the empathy and support we received that day, I will be eternally grateful.

Tuesday Evening

We called my mam and asked her to come and stay with us so we could get up early and go to the hospital the next morning without waking our baby son. Our appointment was for 8.00 am so we wanted to leave at 7.30 am and our little man was not used to getting up before 8.30 am. Mam was happy to help out so we collected her on our way home and brought her back to our house. Then, we picked up the baby from my husband's parents house, where he had spent the day with his Nana and Grandad, and we headed for home.

We felt much more upbeat about things as we got home. We were in good spirits as we ordered Chinese food to be delivered to the house. We had dinner and then we put the little man to bed. We chatted for a while with my mam about the events of the past few days.

My mother had lost a baby before I was born and had often talked about it while I was growing up, so I was familiar with miscarriage. I knew she had been 10 weeks pregnant, had suffered bleeding and cramps and while she was in hospital had lost the baby. She then went on to have a lot of problems when she became pregnant with me, a few months afterwards. She suffered bleeding in early pregnancy and had to stay in bed for several weeks until it ceased. Despite all that, she went on to have a healthy pregnancy and I was born without any complications.

We had some hope and we were feeling optimistic. Even if I knew in my heart it was silly to hope, it was better to hope and feel upbeat than to think about the alternative outcome. My mam was telling us how she had bled for several weeks when she was pregnant with me and I had turned out fine, despite all that. She seemed to know all the right things to say, as she did her best to reassure us. At the time it really did help. Thanks, mam!

We felt much better. We really wanted to believe everything would be OK, so that's what we chose to believe. This little baby, who we had been apprehensive about, was becoming more and more important to us with each passing minute.

Tuesday Night

We decided to go to bed early, as we had an early start ahead of us the next day. We went to bed, chatted for a few minutes and then snuggled up to go to sleep. That was when the pains started. I recognised them immediately. You can never forget labour pains. They are so distinctive and once you have experienced them you will remember them, vividly, for the rest of your life. As I lay there in our bed, I started to curl up into a ball to help ease the pains. "I think I'm in labour," I said to my husband, in a voice of utter disbelief. He started to rub my lower back, which had started aching badly and he was helping me to focus on my breathing.

"I'm losing our baby," I told him. He urged me not to think or speak like that and tried to convince me that it could have been something else. I told him that we needed to go to the hospital straight away. My mam and the baby were asleep in the other rooms and we did not want to wake them, so I got out of bed as quietly as I could and walked towards the bathroom.

When I got into the bathroom there was a "pop". It was exactly like when my waters broke at the end of my first pregnancy but, instead of water, there was blood. There was so much blood. I closed the door over. I don't know why, but I didn't want my husband to see what was happening. I wanted to protect him, I think. Maybe I thought it was bad enough that I had to see it, so I tried to spare him the sight of it. I stood up and there was blood pouring out of me. I don't know how there could have been so much but it seemed like it was never-ending.

Within a few seconds, my husband and my mam were at the door asking me if I was alright. I did not know how to answer. I came out in shreds. I told them our baby was gone. What else could I say? How else could I say it? I knew our baby was gone. My husband went into our bedroom and I could hear him crying. I did not cry then. I was in too much shock and pain to even process any emotions. It was all physical for me at that stage.

As I stood there, the pains came over me again. To be more accurate, they were not pains, they were contractions. I stood against the banister for support and my mam rubbed my back. As I was crouched over, I could hear my husband crying in our bedroom. I was doing my best to hold back the screams I wanted to let out. I wanted to scream for the pain I was in. I wanted to scream over the shock and sadness of what was happening. I kept as quiet as I could and focused on my breathing.

Dave got my overnight bag ready and we made our way downstairs and out to the car. I could barely walk. Dave and my mam had to help me. I was in so much pain. The pains were bad enough but on top of that, I knew there would be no baby at the end of all these painful contractions. It would all be for nothing.

As I left my house I asked my mam if she would clean up the mess I had made in the bathroom. I knew I would not be able to face it when I came home and I did not think Dave would be able to either. The only person in the world who could clean it up was my mam. She is the only person I could have asked to do that. Throughout all the pain and disbelief, I was glad she was there. She gave me some comfort. I also knew she would look after Mitchell for as long as necessary and clean away the reminders of what had happened before I came home.

We drove off and left her there, cleaning up the mess and looking after the baby, who stayed asleep, thankfully. The drive to the hospital was horrible. I thought driving to the hospital when I was in labour on my first baby was challenging but this was a complete nightmare. The contractions were coming hard and fast and I was bleeding quite heavily as well. Apart from the pain and trauma, my husband was fretting. He was trying to drive slowly and carefully but, at the same time, trying to hurry. I knew the baby was gone or going but he still had a shred of hope that it was not gone. I think he was trying to do something in an effort to save us or protect us and the only way he could do that was to get us to the hospital as quickly as he could.

As he drove like a maniac he kept on saying reassuring things to me. I could not believe he still had hope in the midst of what had happened. He is quite optimistic most of the time but this was more optimistic than I could have ever imagined. He was clinging to the faint hope that all was not lost yet. I meekly agreed with him that there may have been a slight chance but in my heart I knew there was none. I just could not face telling him. I thought I could leave that up to the doctors.

We pulled up outside the hospital. It was the second hospital we had visited that afternoon, the hospital where we had Mitchell. They had been so positive earlier that day and we were hoping they would be able to help us and give us some good news about where all the blood was coming from. Well, Dave was hoping, I was already feeling de-feated. Dave rushed around to help me out of the car. There was literally an explosion of blood as I stood up. It was everywhere. As I walked, or to be more accurate, crawled into the hospital, I left a trail behind me. They took me straight into the emergency room and asked my husband to wait outside. There I was lying in a bed in the emer-gency room, in of one of the busiest maternity hos-pitals in the country, by myself, losing my baby.

To make matters even worse, I was lying on a bed with only a flimsy curtain between myself and the woman in the bed next to me. She was 37 weeks pregnant and in labour and I could hear her healthy baby's heartbeat, on a machine, happily beating away, as my baby was leaving me. It was so sad for me to hear life coming into the world right beside me, as my baby was slipping away from me. I felt very conscious of that woman having her baby, in that horrid emergency room. It was bad enough for her that she did not have the time to make it to a delivery suite upstairs but to be laying beside me, a woman losing a baby, must not have been very pleasant for her. Giving birth and meeting your baby for the first time should be a joyous occasion and I did not want to put a cloud over that experience for her, by crying out over the baby I was losing. So I tried to be as quiet as I could.

I also tried to be quiet for the other mothers-to-be who were around me, in that room. It was a nightmare because the emergency room does not have any cubicles; there are only curtains between the patients, which mean everyone knows what is going on beside them. No matter how quiet I tried to be, everyone knew I was losing my baby because I was sobbing and the nurses were talking about me, outside my curtain, wondering whether or not I would need a D&C afterwards. There was no such thing as privacy in that emergency room. I hope someday they can invest in something other than curtains so the apprehensive and sometimes terrified women do not have to hear everything going on around them.

As I lay there, sobbing quietly and breathing through the contractions to the best of my ability, without any pain relief or my husband's hand to squeeze, one of the nurses came over to me and told me that the doctor would be coming soon. It was probably only a few minutes but it seemed like a long time had passed when he finally came to see me. He was a small man, in scrubs. He seemed to be visiting all of the beds in the emergency room and because I was not an "emergency", I was one of the last he came to see. I was lying there, having strong contractions and bleeding very heavily, when he came in to examine me. I never imagined there could be contractions so strong or with so much blood at twelve weeks. I was in so much pain. I was also in shock about how it was happening. I had no idea I would go through something like this. When he examined me, he confirmed that I was in labour and that I was, in fact, losing my baby. I was devastated. Even though I knew it before he told me, there is something so final and definite about a doctor's diagnosis, which made it all very real.

I asked him to get my husband and I also asked for some pain relief. I did not care about all the yoga breathing that had gotten me through the labour and birth first time around. At least that time I knew I would be getting a baby at the end of it all. This time, I knew I would not be meeting my little baby and I just wanted to get away from all the pain. I wanted to be asleep. How could they leave me to go through it, by myself, without any pain relief, especially as I knew there would be no big reward at the end of all that pushing? The doctor said he would come back to me with some pain relief soon and then he told me that my husband would not be allowed in to me – hospital policy! I protested but he explained that no husbands are allowed into the emergency room unless a baby is actually being born. In hindsight, I could have protested that I was in labour and that I was, technically, giving birth but at the time I was so confused and in so much pain I did not have the energy to think of anything like that. With that, he was gone and I was left by myself again, breathing through the very strong contractions and fighting the uncontrollable urge I had to wail and scream.

When we had arrived at the hospital that night, I was (probably foolishly) clinging on to some shred of hope that all was not lost, that, by some chance, our baby was still growing inside of me and that the blood was a result of some other, treatable, pregnancy problem. I know now that it was wishful thinking on my part but it was much easier than the awful truth of what was really happening. I guess because Dave had been so optimistic and he had been trying to convince me that all hope was not lost, I almost believed it – for a short while anyway.

I could not help but feel sorry for myself. How could this be happening to me? I had a perfectly healthy pregnancy first time round. We had a beautiful, healthy, clever little boy at home. This was not supposed to happen. I never expected this and I was not at all prepared for it. As I thought about what was happening, I felt cheated. I did not appreciate the baby as much as I could have while I was pregnant and now I was being robbed of ever knowing this little baby.

Those thoughts did not last long because the contractions were coming so fast and were getting very strong, so I had to put all my energy into getting through them. There was no sign of the doctor with the pain relief. I begged for it. I wanted to be asleep. I could not bear the thought of going through labour and not getting a healthy baby at the end of it all. I wanted someone to inject me with some sleep-inducing drug, so that when I woke up, it would all be over. The nurses told me to focus on my breathing and that would enable me to get through it. I think if Dave had been with me I would have coped so much better but being left on my own to go through the labour was something I did not feel able to do.

I begged them to let my husband in. They just kept telling me that hospital policy is that no husbands or partners are allowed in the emergency room (unless a baby is being born in a hurry) so we could not be together.

I was in labour, by myself, with nobody to hold my hand and help me through it. I was without pain relief, at a time when all the yoga breathing in the world could not help me. I was losing my baby and my husband was not allowed to be with me. I will never understand that policy. Gone are the days when women have to go through all the pregnancy and birth by themselves – husbands and partners can even cut the umbilical cord when a baby is born nowadays – but having a husband or partner when you are losing a baby is not allowed. It is an awful policy and it is so very, very wrong. I will never get over that. In hindsight I wish I had protested more and then, perhaps, they would have let him in. However, at the time I could hardly focus on anything other than the pain, so I did not think about causing a fuss over it.

I was in a great deal of pain and distress but I also wanted to know how my husband was doing. I knew he was outside, thinking the worst, after what had happened in the house and in the car on the way to the hospital. I asked a nurse to check on him for me and let me know how he was. As she left, she told me to concentrate on my breathing. She came back and told me that he was sitting in the waiting area, with his head in his hands. I felt even worse. He was outside, distressed, upset and waiting for an update on the baby and I was inside, worrying about him, while I was going through the worst ordeal of my life. I sometimes wish she had lied to me. Perhaps she did not need to tell me he was sitting there, with his head in his hands?

After a while the doctor came in to check on me again. I begged and pleaded with them to let my husband in. They said they would see what they could do. In the meantime, they asked me to take a deep breath and give a big push. I tried but nothing happened. I could hear the doctor saying to the nurse that there was a blockage, where all the blood had gathered. She went away and got a hook-like instrument and he inserted this inside me and "unblocked" the birth canal. There was a huge rush of blood but, horrifically, there were lots of lumps in the blood. I felt some relief, as I had been trying to push it out myself but could not. However, when I saw what had come out, I became very upset – hysterical is probably a better description. I wanted to know if my baby was in with all that blood. They whisked away everything, so I could not really see. They told me they would have to send it all up to the laboratory for examination.

I was left there, empty, broken and alone. I had never felt more alone in my life. As I could hear the heartbeats of the healthy babies who were soon to be born in the room around me, I was acutely aware that there was no longer a little baby inside me. I felt cold and shattered. Finally, they gave me some pain relief. It was probably to put me asleep because I had been through the worst of it at that stage. I don't even remember what it was. All I know is it made me feel numb – or perhaps I had just gone into shock. I don't know. I remember that, after the drug, the pain was less and the bleeding was less. Soon after, I could hear the nurse on the phone asking someone upstairs to get a bed ready for me. She told them I had suffered a "complete miscarriage" and had been given some pain relief, which would probably send me off into a good night's sleep. Therefore, they wanted to get me up to the ward and settled as soon as possible.

Early Hours of Wednesday 26th February

The nurse came over and told me they would be bringing me upstairs into a ward very soon. I asked her when I would be able to see my husband. She told me to wait another minute and then I would be able to see him. She put me in a wheelchair and wheeled me out of the emergency room.

He was sitting there quietly, waiting for me to come out. I will never forget the look on his face. They had not actually told him that the baby was gone, so I had to confirm it for him. I did not need to speak; he could see it all in my face. That was harder than the labour, having to confirm that to Dave. We looked at each other and we both broke down and cried. I uttered something about being sorry and I cannot quite remember what he said to me but I know he was trying to comfort me. He told me it was not my fault but he was crumbling too. It was an overwhelming feeling of hopelessness and sadness and we were both enveloped in it.

They wheeled me up to the ward. Dave walked beside me, touching me and holding my hand, trying to comfort me in some way. Once we reached the room, they put me into the bed. I needed some help because the drugs had started to kick in. I was exhausted from the labour and with the drugs they had given me; I was starting to feel groggy and sleepy. I am so grateful that I was drugged. I knew there was a world of pain waiting for me but I was nowhere near being ready to face it. Instead I had the luxury of a numbing feeling washing over me, helping block out that pain. I did not want to know about that pain. I wanted to bury it and not deal with it. It was too awful to be true. My baby was dead. My little angel was gone. All that was left was a hollow, empty feeling and I did not want to know about it. For one night, I would sleep soundly from whatever drug they gave me. I could pretend I did not have to deal with it. I could drift off into a dreamless sleep and not worry about the reality of it all, at least until the next day anyway.

I remember so clearly lying there, feeling quite peaceful. It was so strange. I had just been through a nightmare that, unfortunately for me, was not really a nightmare, it was a harsh reality. I had just lost my baby. Still, I remember feeling floaty and light-headed.

That was all about to change. I had a sudden urge to pee. As I stood up to go to the bathroom I felt dizzy. I really thought that most of it had to be gone at that stage but I was wrong. I had been amazed at the amount of it and now as I got up out of the bed, I could feel it gathering again. I went into the toilets. I think I rushed but I was starting to feel really groggy, so I probably just walked slowly.

I went into the cubicle and all of a sudden there was another "pop". Another huge amount of blood, and something else, just poured out of me. I screamed. I thought it was my baby, lying there on the floor. There was something in the middle of all the blood.

The nurse, who had helped me to the toilet, was waiting outside for me. When she heard me scream, she rushed in and scooped it all up off the floor and took it away for analysis. I asked her if that was my baby I had seen and she reassured me that it was not. She told me it was just tissue from the placenta and that the baby was definitely well gone at this stage.

I wished I could have seen my baby. I wanted to say sorry for not cherishing him or her more than I had. I wanted to say goodbye. I felt cheated that he or she was just robbed from me so suddenly. It seemed so unfair. On top of those feelings, I was thinking about the labour and the utensils they had used to help me deliver. I could not help but think that the baby had been harmed on his or her way out by the utensils the doctor had used to "unclog" me. That was so hurtful to think about. It was bad enough that my baby was gone but I wanted to think that he or she had just slipped away peacefully. Instead, all I could think about was that the baby was damaged and pulled at during the delivery.

I knew I was being irrational. The baby was so small that we probably would not have seen it in the midst of all the blood and tissue, but I was just bordering on going crazy at that stage, especially after the bathroom incident.

Soon I was back in bed, with my husband holding my hand and urging me to go off to sleep. I was feeling very tired, after all I had been through. Labour itself is hard enough, without adding the trauma of losing a baby, so I was completely shattered. That, added to the drugs, had me ready for sleep.

I held my husband's hand and made him promise not to leave me until I was definitely asleep. I had been alone for so much of that night and I wanted him to be with me until I was gone into a sleep and away from the horror of what had happened. He stayed with me for what seemed like a long time and eventually, somewhere in the early hours of the morning, I fell asleep.

When I woke up it was all very hazy. I felt tired and groggy and for a few seconds I did not quite know what was going on. Then reality hit me. Reality, free from drugs, hit me. It was too awful to be real. I could not bear to think about it. The nurse came in and asked me how I was feeling. I am not sure if I answered her, I just wanted to go home. I wanted to be away from the place where this tragedy had happened. I wanted to be at home, in my own bed, where I could sleep and forget about it all for a while. I wanted to go home and kiss my baby boy. I knew I was so lucky to have a baby at home. Even though I knew he could not fill the void that had been left in me, I still wanted to kiss and cuddle him and tell him how much I loved him. I wanted to be at home with my husband. I hated that we had been separated and I wanted to be back home, with him and my son and nobody else.

I did not want to see or talk to anyone else. I did not want to have to talk about it because if I had to talk about it then I would have to deal with it.

She asked me to go with her to the room across the hall for an ultrasound scan to check whether or not I had suffered a complete miscarriage. She started the scan and told me she was looking for anything left inside. If there was anything left, she told me I might need an operation to remove it. That was a horrible thought. I had been through three hours of labour and was still bleeding what seemed like an endless river of blood, so I was hoping that everything was "gone". I was devastated that it was gone but when she mentioned a D&C, I was suddenly hoping that it was all gone. In truth, there was a very small part of me that longed for the D&C procedure, just so I could have the anaesthetic. I almost wanted to be put to sleep and have the D&C, or as it's also known, ERPC surgery, that would clean out my womb for me, so I could escape from the reality of the situation. Having the procedure and being put to sleep would mean I could block it all out for a few more hours and that was a tempting thought at the time. It would allow me to be free, for a little longer, from the emotional nightmare that awaited me. I know that makes no sense but I would have done almost anything at that point to go into a deep sleep where I would not dream or think about anything for a few more hours . . .

After the scan the nurse brought me back to my bed. She was very kind; she said some comforting things to me. She held my hand and told me it was just nature's way of not letting the pregnancy progress. She also told me that it looked like I would not need a D&C after all, but that the doctor would have the final say on that.

Soon after, the doctor came to see me. He said he had some good news (as if there is ever good news at a time like that). He confirmed that because I had suffered a complete miscarriage, I would not need to have a D&C procedure. It meant I could go home that morning. I was relieved because, in the face of it, I did not want to be put under anaesthetic so they could clean out my womb for me. There was some comfort in knowing that was not necessary. I would have liked the anaesthetic, but not the rest of it.

As I lay there, waiting for my husband to come in to get me, I remember thinking how nature can be so efficient. My body had totally rejected the baby and did everything possible to get rid of the baby and everything associated with it. I would soon dread the words that most people would say to me – "It was not meant to be and it was nature's way of making sure it didn't happen" – but it's true.

It was my body's way of not letting it happen. There was something wrong and because of whatever defect it was, my baby was gone.

As I was preparing to leave, the nurse mentioned something to me about a counselling service at the hospital. I did not really hear what she was saying but I vaguely remember her telling me that I could book an appointment with the hospital counsellor if I felt I needed it. I was so eager to just get out of there that I did not really take it in at the time. She left some information about it and said I should take it home with me. I was so numb I hardly knew what she was talking about but I put the information into my bag anyway. Just in case.

I was ready to go home and sat there waiting for my husband. He came in and it was like it had all just happened at that moment. The hurt in his face brought it all rushing to the front of my mind again and I felt shattered. So many emotions ripped through me as I looked into his eyes. I felt sad for him; I knew he was devastated. I felt sad that my baby was gone. I felt guilty that I had not cherished the baby more when he or she was still with me. Once again, I chastised myself for spending more time thinking about being pregnant than I did thinking about our little baby – I sorely regretted that. I felt like I was being punished.

Despite the heartache I was going through, I also felt somewhat relieved. It had been an unbelievably tough week both emotionally and physically and I was glad it was finally over – at least in one way. I knew the emotional trauma was just beginning but at least physically I was over the worst. It had been horrific and I was somewhat relieved I was over that part of the ordeal. All these thoughts flooded my head as I thought to myself that I needed to get a grip, I was heading home to see my baby son and I needed to be strong for him.

Dave's recollections . . .

AS WE GOT INTO MONTH TWO of the pregnancy (and once the young lad was asleep) I always enjoyed lying close to Siobhán in bed, knowing that I was only inches away from my little baby. It just made me feel closer to the baby in psychological terms; I felt like somehow I was protecting the little one.

The day we first noticed the blood was very tough; I felt totally useless. I remember Siobhán getting very upset. She had a look of defeat on her face and all I could think was to try and keep her calm, so at least then the baby would be calm; that was my rationale at that point. I wanted to make her laugh or smile or whatever . . . anything just to make sure she was happy and then hopefully, this would rub off on the baby and the baby would be happy too. I was so desperate to feel useful because I felt like it was out of my hands. Despite trying to be positive, at the back of my mind I felt that something bad was happening.

As the days of that awful week went by, I tried my best to protect and comfort Siobhan, but how could I protect her from the doctors who were supposed to be looking after her? I'll never forget when the doctor who was performing the scan uttered the words, "It probably just has not happened yet". For a second I was sure he could not actually have said those words. Then my brain thought about it and I realised he had; the words were still in the air, "It probably just has not happened yet". I could feel my fists tighten, and total rage coming over me. "Who the FUCK do you think you are?" flashed through my mind. I wanted to obliterate this idiot; but I stopped for a second, looked at my defeated wife and retreated. It was not the time and certainly not the place for anger or aggression. What good would a reaction like that have done anyway?

I remember the night it happened so clearly. I had my arm around Siobhán's belly. We were lying very close together and somehow I felt that maybe, even then, I could save my baby. But then it happened. No matter what I did, the situation was out of my control. I could not help her. I rubbed her back but she crawled out of the bed, away from me. I said comforting things but she could not be comforted. I felt totally helpless. There was nothing I could do. As a man, I felt desperately powerless. I could not stop it.

When she came out of the bathroom, ghost-like, and told me that she had lost our baby, I couldn't believe it. No; she was wrong; she had to be wrong; this couldn't happen to our baby, not to my baby? I went into our room to get her pre-packed case and it hit me: our baby was slipping away. Then, suddenly, the tears started flowing down my face. It had been a while since I had cried like that, not since the birth of our son, but there I was, once again, crying uncontrollably. I knew I had to get it together, at least for Siobhán's sake. I pulled myself together and convinced myself that there might still be some hope.

As crazy as it sounds, something told me the baby was still with us and as I was driving erratically toward the hospital, I tried to convince Siobhán that everything would be OK. As we parked, a group of girls walked by, obviously out for the night. They were laughing and joking, as our world was collapsing around us, and I thought to myself that Siobhán had been just like one of them, carefree and having fun, only two years ago. But not at that moment. There and then, she was broken. She looked like a shell of herself and there was nothing I could do to fix her.

When we walked from the car into the hospital I could see a trail of blood behind Siobhán; I did everything I could to make sure she didn't see it. She was brought into the ER instantly and I had to wait outside, to give our details. I thought that, once I was finished, I would be able to join my wife. As I approached the ER, a nurse said to me, "No, you

cannot go in there, you sit over there and we'll look
after your wife!" Like a fool, I did what I was told
and sat down. My mind was racing. The situation
was completely out of my control. There was nothing I could do and on top of that, I was not allowed
to be with my wife, at a time when we needed to be
together. As anyone who knows me will testify, I
rarely do what I'm told to do, but I just sat there. I
must have been in shock because I simply sat there
quietly, waiting for the nurses to tell me what was
going on. I guess I figured that, because I was in a
hospital, they knew better than I did. I suppose I
thought that they knew what they were doing and
if a doctor said we should do something then we
should . . . obey.

I was left sitting there, alone. Nobody came over
to tell me anything. My wife was in an emergency
room, losing our baby, and I had to sit there by myself. Every emotion was passing over me: anger,
sadness, stupidity, anger, sadness. How was
Siobhán? How was my baby? After about an hour I
went up to the desk to ask about my wife and baby.
At one stage, I had to turn away and fight back the
tears, only to see everyone in the waiting room staring at me. I found myself standing at the reception
desk, screaming crying, just wanting to know what
the fuck was going on. I was told they would check
for me and that I would be better off sitting down,
and very coolly the girl returned to her computer.

As I sat down again and composed myself I could see a small girl with her dad. They had found themselves sitting in that waiting room, probably for something serious too. Amazingly, I found myself playing peek-a-boo with the little girl, who was only two or three years old; what did she know? Her dad gave me an appreciative nod, as I returned to my hell of waiting. Nobody came to tell me what was happening. I had to wait until my wife was wheeled out in a wheelchair, and still I clung to the smallest shred of hope, although once I looked in Siobhán's distant eyes, I knew.

The nurse wheeled Siobhán out and then they finally told me that my wife had a miscarriage; why had it taken so long for me to be told? They did not seem to realise that dads suffer too at times like that. They had not considered me at all. They did not give me updates on what was happening. They would not let me in to see Siobhán, despite the fact that she was in labour by herself. They made me feel totally useless and like it was not any of my business to know what was happening. In hindsight, I should have protested or done or said something, instead of just sitting there quietly but at the time I just did not know what to do.

We got into the lift to go upstairs. Siobhán was subdued, staring into space. She looked so frail and weak. The nurse was quiet. Amid the silence, it finally dawned on me that our baby was gone. We got into the ward and I helped Siobhán into bed.

She was groggy from the drugs but even so, I
wanted to comfort her and stay with her until she
was asleep. This was the first time I had felt useful
since we had arrived at the hospital and I was going
to do everything I could to make sure she was as
comfortable as possible.

Siobhán needed to go to the bathroom and the
nurse said she would go with her. I sat there at her
bedside by myself, as the plans and dreams I had
for the baby unravelled in my head. I was devastated but determined to stay strong for Siobhán.

When she came back from the bathroom she
looked even worse than before. She told me what
had happened. The nurse assured me it was "normal" for this to happen as we helped Siobhán into
bed. She said that sleep would be the best thing for
her now and urged her to go to sleep.

Soon after we got her into bed, and once I had
managed to calm her down after the incident in the
bathroom, she fell asleep and I was advised to go
home and get some rest too. As I was leaving, I
could not help but remember the last time I had left
that hospital, after the birth of Mitchell. That time, I
bounced down the stairs, hopped through reception
with a huge smile on my face after witnessing the
birth of my baby boy but this time I dragged myself
out the door, my shoulders drooped, my neck sore,
my legs weak and my heart very heavy. I was shattered.

I got into the car and started driving. I was in a trance; had all of that just happened, was my baby really dead? For some reason I needed to listen to my favourite song. I pushed in the CD, pressed track number three and listened to the first line, "Is it getting better? Or do you feel the same?" I realised I would never feel the same again, I was enveloped in emptiness and then hysterical crying followed. I managed to pull over off the road and I sat there for half an hour, screaming crying. I could not help but wonder why had this happened to us? Why us? Why?

I eventually got home. It must have been 4.00 am and Siobhán's mam came downstairs when I walked in. I fell onto the floor. She did not need to ask me; she just knew. She had been through losing a baby herself and so she just came over to me and put her arms around me. She did her best to comfort me but I could not be consoled. We went into the kitchen and I just motioned for a cigarette (I'd been off them for a year and a half), we had our smoke and I explained what had happened.

Soon after, I went up to bed. I lay there, just replaying the previous hours' events, over and over in my head. Eventually I must have fallen asleep, as I remember waking up and instantly returning to hell.

It was still early in the morning when I got ready, peeked at my sleeping son through his door, thanked God for him and went back to the hospital. As I walked into the ward and looked at my wife, I could not believe how she looked. She is normally the kind of person with a big smile, someone who lights up any room she's in, but she was just lying there motionless. She seemed to be a million miles away. I've never seen her look so defeated. She was shredded. I tried my best to comfort her but it seemed in vain; she – we – just wanted to get out of there. While Siobhán was waiting for the doctor to see her, before she could be discharged, we decided to ring those closest to us to tell them our sad news.

I knew Siobhán could not make those calls; she did not want to talk to any one, so I had to do it. It was tough. I had to get over my grief to be strong and calm on the phone. As much as we were upset that we had lost our baby, I knew the grandparents and aunts and uncles would be sad too, so I put my tears on hold until I was finished on the phone. I tried to be strong for Siobhán and for those close to us.

When I got back up to Siobhán it was time to go home. The drive was understandably hard for the two of us. It was filled with small talk: "How's Mitchell?" "Do you think he'll understand?" "Who did you get to speak to?" "Did you leave a message for the people we could not get through to?" We talked about everything except the one thing we should have been talking about. Most importantly, even though we were brushing over the issue, we had to be there for each other.

Chapter 3

The Aftermath

Siobhán's recollections . . .

WE LEFT THE HOSPITAL. I honestly do not remember actually walking out of the hospital, or getting into the car, or being driven home. I have absolutely no memory of any of that. I must have been in a daydream. I cannot remember one second of it. All I remember is sitting on the hospital bed, ready to go, and then pulling up in the driveway of our house.

My mam was there minding Mitchell but I did not feel up to facing her. It's so strange. My mam and I are very close. She suffered a miscarriage herself, so she should have been the one person I wanted to see but I did not want to. I don't know why. When I walked into the house she threw her arms open and tried to hug me. I literally pushed her away and just muttered that I was fine. I did not cry one tear, while she had tears running down her face. I think I hurt her so much in that moment, but

I was so afraid to actually cry. I was terrified that if I let her hug me and I let my emotions out, then perhaps I would never stop crying. I brushed past her and picked up my baby boy. I gave him lots of hugs and cuddles but I don't think I cried at all that morning. It is so hazy to me.

Dave made me some breakfast and ushered me up to bed. I know he and my mam were terribly worried about me, so they just did what they thought was best. First they made me a cup of tea and some breakfast and then they tried to get me to go to sleep. As we all know in Ireland, if you're not well, you have to have a nice cup of tea first and then a lie down – and then you'll feel much better. It did not work. There are not enough cups of tea in the world to help with the pain of losing a baby.

I went to bed. I actually fell asleep. I did not think I would or could after what had happened and with all the thoughts flying around my head but sheer exhaustion got the better of me and I fell into a restless sleep.

That afternoon I woke up. It was so horrible waking up because for a couple of seconds I thought I was still pregnant and had maybe just been having a lie-down, but then reality slapped me in the face and the horror of what had happened hit me again. Sleep was lovely but waking up was aw-ful. I wanted to stay asleep forever – at least on that first day when the pain was so raw.

I went downstairs to a very cautious husband and a very protective mother. They both wanted so much to help me and I just wanted them to leave me alone. That day is such a blur to me but I do remember that my dad came to collect my mam that afternoon and he brought my little sisters, Denise and Kate, who were aged 10 and 12 at the time, with him.

I have always been very close to my siblings and I had decided that I wanted to tell them the sad news myself. My mam offered to do it and so did my husband, but I wanted to give them the truth, straight from me. They arrived and I called them into the sitting room. They looked very anxious as we sat them down. My mam and dad kept our son in the other room, so Dave and I could tell them what had happened.

We told them that the baby had not been growing properly and because of this, had died. We explained that the baby was not hurt in any way but that he or she slipped away and that he or she was now a little angel up in heaven. They were very sad but very brave and I was glad I had told them myself. Their questions, which were so blunt, made it easier to tell them than to tell an adult. There is something so refreshingly straight about a child asking questions; they just asked what they wanted to know and we just answered. Simple.

My dad knew what had happened before he arrived at the house and when he came in, he put a supportive arm around me. I appreciated the gesture but I did not want anyone near me or reassuring me, so I pulled away from him as well. I just could not handle it, so I stayed away from everyone, as much as I could.

Soon afterwards they left and then it was just the three of us. The phone rang a lot that day and I let Dave answer it. I did not want to talk to anyone about it. I went to bed early that night hoping that I would feel better after a good night's sleep.

The next morning brought the same horror. I woke up, felt fine and then, after just a few seconds, I felt empty again. I turned to my husband and told him that I did not want to get up. I did not want to do anything. I wanted to stay in bed and feel sorry for myself. However, soon after, Mitchell woke up in the next room and we had to get up. It's probably just as well he did wake up because he stopped me from brooding all morning in bed. We had to get him up, feed him, wash him, dress him and play with him.

I am very grateful that we had a little boy at home because he was exactly what we needed at that time. He made us realise that no matter what happens, life goes on and you need to deal with it. You cannot close the curtains and pretend it's not out there, because it is. Whenever he laughed or did something funny that day, it seemed to be the most special thing he had ever done. I guess I had a new-found appreciation for how wonderful he was and I wanted to cherish him more than I ever had.

I could not help but think about how awful it must have been for my mam when she lost her baby. She had suffered a miscarriage on her first pregnancy, so she did not have any baby to go home to. That must have been so tough. She often spoke of her fears that she might never be able to conceive. She was beside herself with worry that she would never become pregnant again. Luckily for her, she went on to have healthy babies, as do most women who suffer a miscarriage, but as I looked lovingly at my child, it struck me that it must be extra difficult to suffer a miscarriage on a first pregnancy.

With that in mind, I was showering Mitchell with extra cuddles and kisses. As if he knew there was something wrong, he allowed me to hold him for ages in those first few days. He was a very active ten-month-old at that stage and was able to walk (and almost run) around the furniture and also loved to play on the floor with his toys but when we lost the baby and I was so sad, he seemed to sense I needed extra time with him. It's amazing how babies can pick up on our mood; even at that age he knew to let me cuddle him for hours on end.

He was the only person I felt happy around. Family and friends, even my own mother who had been through the horror of losing a baby herself, could not make me feel any better. This little guy,

who was not yet fully able to walk or talk, was my
main source of comfort. He must have been wondering why he was getting so many cuddles from
his mammy.

Even my husband was getting on my nerves.
Dave was so upset and quite often he would break
down and cry. I am appalled to admit that I was
getting annoyed with all his crying. It sounds so
terrible when I admit it like that, but it's the truth. I
appreciate a man who is able to show his emotions
but at that time, I wished he could have been one of
those men who just do not cry. I know it's much
better when a person can let their emotions out,
rather than bottle them up inside and I should have
been relieved that he was able to let it out like that;
but honestly, I wanted to tell him just to stop all his
crying and get on with things. I could not bring
myself to actually say that to him, so I sulked away
quietly to myself.

For some reason, I was frustrated with him for
being so upset. Perhaps I was really upset that he
was showing it so readily because I could not – or
would not. I know now that he was just doing what
was right for him. Those emotions had to come out
of him and he was letting them. Unlike him, I was
blocking all the pain away, deep down inside, and
far from surfacing. I was tucking it away in the back
of my mind, where I would not have to deal with it.
As far as I was concerned, I *had* dealt with it and
that was that. Life goes on and I was getting on with

things. That was the only way I could cope at that time. I suppose I should have known that it would all have to come out at some stage but for that time, I was happy to pretend I was fine, getting on with the day-to-day things and not talking about it.

A few days after the baby was gone, the phone started ringing and the cards started coming in the post. I was annoyed when anyone sent a card or phoned to see how I was but at the same time, I was even more annoyed at anyone who did not phone or send a card. I think I just wanted to take my anger out on anyone I could and I was picking at any excuse to do so. I read the cards and I put them away. I spoke to the callers and was devoid of emotion as they tried not to cry on the other end of the phone. Some people, like my friend Emma and aunt Christine, were so upset when they called that they were on the verge of tears and I found myself reassuring them that I was fine and it was just nature's way of not letting this little baby into the world.

It seems crazy now that I was reassuring *them* but such was my denial that I was able to be practical about the whole situation. I was able to tell them, without breaking down or shedding one little tear, that my baby was not meant to be and that it was probably for the best. I was perfectly able to talk and reassure them but they were shaky, nervous and upset when talking to me. I guess they expected me to be a wreck, constantly crying, and they got quite a shock when they heard me being so matter-of-fact on the other end of the phone. I was actually a bit annoyed at them too for almost crying when they were talking to me. In my mind I thought I was being strong and I expected everyone else to be strong too. It just did not occur to me that they would be upset and would cry about it – because I was choosing not to deal with it at that time. In my mind, they did not have the right to cry; that was my right and I chose not to, so they should have followed suit and kept their sadness away from me. Denial – it's a dangerous state of mind.

Somewhere in my mind I knew it was perfectly acceptable for the people close to Dave and me to be upset and to cry when they spoke to us about our loss but I just wanted to tell them all to get a grip. If I was not breaking down crying all the time, then why should everyone else be? It was my baby and I was not crying about it, so why should they be sobbing down the phone to me about it?

As I write this now I realise how completely deluded I was. Never was there a person in so much denial of their feelings. I was actually happy when the phone did not ring, so I would not have to hear other people tell me how sad they were for us over what had happened. It's awful to admit that but it's true. I would sometimes take a call from a friend or relative and I would roll my eyes, in anticipation of getting them off the phone as soon as possible. I was in no mood to comfort anyone else when I thought I was over it. I expected everyone else to be over it too. That's why my husband was annoying me so much. He was clearly not over it and it was annoying me that I had to reassure him. I wanted to get past it and not talk about it.

It was not just Dave; I did not want to talk about it with anyone. I did not want other people to talk about it either. It was my business and I did not want to be the subject for local gossip. Even if people were genuinely offering their condolences, I did not want to accept them. I did not want anyone talking about me or my baby, no matter what context it was in. I remember being particularly angry at my mam when she told me that she had told her friends at work about how sad she was because we had lost the baby. Imagine it, the craziness of it: I was annoyed at her for being upset about losing her grandchild.

It makes no sense but that's what was happening to me. I was turning into a nightmare. I had no patience at all. Everything and everyone was annoying me. I was not crying or getting upset like my husband. Oh no, I was taking it out on the people who love me, the people who were trying to help me.

After a few weeks of my dark moods, it did not come as much of a shock when my husband suggested, or should I say persuaded, me to make an appointment with the hospital counsellor. I argued with him that I did not "need" to see the hospital counsellor. I protested and said I did not need to go but after much discussion and the realisation that perhaps it was not healthy that he had been the only one in our house crying about it, I succumbed and reluctantly agreed to go.

I called the hospital and made the appointment. (The appointment was for me only, the counselling service was not offered to Dave.) I went to see her exactly one month after the baby had died. I was so matter of fact about it. I got up and got dressed. I put on some make-up, including mascara, because I was damn sure that I would not be doing any crying that day. I dropped the little man off to his Nana's house and headed up to the hospital for my appointment. I went in, sat down and started reading a magazine. I was more interested in which handbag went with which shoes that season than why I was really there. I was sitting there, happily catching up on all the ce-lebrity gossip, when the counsellor finally called me into her office.

I went in and sat down. I was so determined not to cry. I still cannot understand my absolute resis-tance to letting my guard down. I am the type of person who cries at soppy books and films but there I was, having lost my baby, determined not to cry about it. I thought I was handling everything very well and that my husband was a big softie . . . until I started talking that day with the counsellor. She led me into a very cramped, messy office and introduced herself. She told me she had worked upstairs in a different department but she needed to cut back on her hours, so she had been transferred to counselling. I'm not sure if she was a qualified counsellor. She was not very professional and she did talk about herself quite a bit, which I would not have expected a professional counsellor to do, but she was a very nice lady and she definitely did make me feel better. She let me tell her all about how it had happened. From the first spot of blood, right through to the awful, horrific end, three days later. She let me speak. She did not interrupt with well-wishing comments or words of advice or suggestions that I "could always have another baby". (As if having another baby can ever, ever, replace a lost baby. It cannot. Nothing can ever replace losing a baby, so that comment is really not helpful when you've lost a baby and unfortunately, it's the one that's said most.)

I told her all about how I was alone in the emergency room when I was in labour and how awful it was that my husband had to wait outside. It occurred to me that I was *very* angry about that. I was not angry at the people who called me or sent me cards or wished me well (even though I was taking it out on them). I was angry at the hospital for not letting my husband in to be with me, when I was going through that ordeal. I was angry and it actually gave me a sense of relief to admit that out loud. I started to feel a bit better that I was finally talking about that. It felt good to complain out loud. It was

a start. I was talking about it and that was something positive.

I spent an hour with her and she asked me a lot
of questions and I honestly did feel much better by
the end of it. During our session she gave me a
handout with a list of "normal emotions" listed on
it. These were the emotions people often experienced after a loss, such as a miscarriage. It was a
long list and as I read down through it, I was surprised by all the emotions on there. Anger, despair,
depression, irritability, guilt . . . the list was very
long and I was comforted to see some of the emotions I had been feeling on there. As much as I hate
to categorise myself, I felt a bit better that my re-
sponses were somewhat "normal".

Before I left, I got some homework! She urged
me to keep a diary. She suggested I write into it
every night and that no matter how awful the day
had been, the rule was that I had to write two good
things that had happened that day, at the end of
each page. I could do that, I thought. I loved writing and I could always find something good in each
day to write at the end of the page. So I agreed to
buy a little diary on my way home.

The next bit of homework was to do something
nice for myself and my husband. She asked me not
to go and collect my son straight away. She suggested that I ask his Nana if she would be able to
keep him for the afternoon, so that I could go off and
buy two presents, one for myself and one for my

husband. She said we deserved a treat after the month we had been through. As a devoted shopaholic, I was delighted to be getting instructions, from a counsellor, to go shopping. I called my mother-in-law as I left the hospital and asked if she could keep my son for a couple more hours. She was only too happy to have him (she is great with him and she loves any excuse to have him for a few hours) and so off I went on the hunt for two pressies.

As I had some time for myself, I decided to go up to the lovely Chocolate Soup Café in Roches Stores for a bowl of hot chocolate. With a ten-month-old keeping me busy all the time I did not get much chance for leisurely coffees anymore, so the thought of a few moment's peace over a hot choccy really appealed to me.

I wandered up the escalator towards the café. I went in and ordered my hot chocolate and a piece of cake. As I was waiting for my order, my husband called me. "Well, how did you get on?" he asked. That was it. That was the straw that broke the camel's back, as the saying goes. That one little question was all it took to send me over the edge. I did not cry in the counsellor's office. I did not cry when I left her office. I had felt emotional but I had decided that morning that I would not be doing any crying that day (oh, how deluded I really was!) and up to that point I had not shed one tear. I had been leaving all the crying to my husband! But then, just as I heard his voice, it all changed. As he tenderly, cautiously asked me how it went, I exploded into tears, right there at the counter. The tears started to fly out of my eyes. It must have looked like something out of a Looney Toons cartoon – you know how, when one of the characters cries, their animated tears fly into the air at great speed. It felt like that. I was inconsolable and quite unable to speak to him and he was getting rather concerned.

As I stood there, balling my eyes out, trying to say something to my husband to stop him fretting about the wailing noises I was making, the girl turned around with my hot chocolate and cake. She just froze and stood there, with my drink in her hand, a stunned look on her face. She looked really uncomfortable and did not know whether to take my order away or put it on my tray. I guess her training did not cover how to deal with inconsolable customers. I could not manage words so I nodded, took out my purse and gestured to her that I still wanted what I had ordered. I eventually managed to gurgle down the phone to my other half – "I'll call you back in a few minutes" – who must have been up the walls with worry at that stage. I put the phone down and, through my sobs, paid for my goodies.

It's funny that even though the floodgates had just opened and would remain open for quite some time, I still wanted to have my afternoon treat. Some people might have run out of the shop after such a crying session at the counter but I got my tray and walked over to a secluded seat and I sat down. I cried there, in Roches Stores Chocolate Soup Café, for about 40 minutes. In between sobs I managed to sip my drink and nibble away at my cake. I even managed a quick call to my husband, to let him know that I was OK and reassured him that I did not need to be committed, not just yet.

In a strange way it was one of the most pleasant afternoons I have ever had. I felt so relieved. A huge weight was being lifted off my shoulders. All the tension and stress I had been keeping locked away was finally being let out and it felt good. It was as if a sense of peace was coming over me, as I cried my eyes out in that café. In hindsight I probably should have worn waterproof mascara but I did not really care! So what if my cheeks looked like they had train-tracks painted onto them? So what if people were staring at me and giving me funny glances as I sobbed, sipped, sobbed and nibbled my way through a lot of tears, a very tasty hot chocolate and a big piece of cake? All the emotions inside of me had been locked away and now they were finally being released. And, oh, how they were being released.

After I had cried my eyes out, finished my goodies and cleaned my face as best I could, I browsed around the shops for an hour or two. I picked up some food and wine and was planning to make a special dinner that night. I was able to have a few glasses of wine now that I was no longer pregnant, so I decided it would be a nice treat to relax over a good meal and some wine with my hubby. We might even feel slightly *normal* again.

I picked up Mitchell and headed home. I put the food on and opened the wine. I had everything more or less prepared when my other half walked in. I thought I had cried all the tears a person could cry in one day but, oh no, there were more left in me. As soon as I looked at Dave, they came rushing to the surface again. Once again, I was inconsolable. I could not stop crying. He just hugged me and re-assured me – and for the first time since we had lost our baby, it was me doing all the crying and him doing the comforting.

I think he was relieved that I was actually crying it all out. It was crazy the way I had been bottling it all up, but now at least it was all coming out. Better late than never, I suppose. We put the little man to bed, had a lovely dinner and some wine and I cried my way through the evening. I cried and cried and cried. After we thought I could cry no more, we decided to watch a movie together. I had rented one that day; it was supposed to be a comedy. Well, it was not very funny when one of the characters died because it just served to remind me of our loss and I was off again, crying for Ireland.

The next day, I cried again and the following day and the day after that. For the next month I cried a lot. I was grieving, finally, for the little baby we had lost. I was facing up to the fact that the little life that had been growing inside me was now gone and would be gone forever. I was feeling the loss in a very profound way. I was devastated.

I also started to write into a diary every night, as the counsellor had recommended. It was a very therapeutic exercise. If I was mad or sad about something, I wrote it down. It was like a de-stressing mechanism. It enabled me to get things off my chest, even if it was only on paper. Still, it made me feel better and it was a good outlet for all the emotions I was feeling, so that cannot be bad. (I would recommend keeping a diary to anyone who has suffered a loss. Write down what happened during the day and most importantly, end your diary entry with two positive things that happened that day. That will ensure you think about the good things before you nod off to sleep. As time goes by, your pain will become more bearable and the diary entries will become more positive.)

I remember my friend Rhona came to visit me that weekend. She brought me a bunch of my favourite flowers, peach tulips, and some cake. When I opened the door she handed me the flowers and gave me a big hug. (She gives the best hugs in the world; she just makes you feel so special and loved when she pulls you in for one of her trademark hugs.) It was the first time I felt comfortable with a visitor and I wanted to sit down and talk about it with her over a cup of tea or, as it turned out, about three pots of tea. She was the first person to ask me

really direct questions about how it had all happened and it was one of the first times I felt comfortable actually answering those questions. I remember it so vividly. She asked me everything and
it felt good to talk about it. I guess seeing the counsellor and writing in my diary every night was
helping. I felt more open about it and was not getting annoyed or angry anymore. I wanted to talk
about it now. It was awful but it *had* happened and
there was no denying it anymore.

Until that point I did not really talk to anyone
about it but I was feeling different now. I answered
every question she asked me and we talked for
most of the afternoon. It was like a dose of therapy.
I felt much better after it, like another burden had
been lifted off my shoulders. I realised that talking
about it openly, and not being afraid to share my
pain with others, was much better, for me and for
them. My family and friends had wanted to help
me but I had not been letting them until that point
but I knew that was all about to change after that
afternoon. I was no longer afraid to let people ask
me about it and that was certainly a move in the
right direction.

I wanted to get away for a few days so I booked
a weekend away with my mam. I was planning to
visit my sister, Sabrina, in Jersey. We had always
been very close and I had not seen her since we had
lost the baby, so I wanted to talk to her about it. We
headed off for our weekend a few weeks after I had

first seen the counsellor. I was feeling much better about things and was able to talk about it more openly now, so I felt I would be able to spend a few days away and genuinely relax and enjoy myself. I was glad my mam was coming with me. She was a pillar of support for me through that whole time. She was the one person I was able to talk to in detail about it because she had been through losing a baby herself.

We spent some time shopping and having leisurely lunches and it was all very nice and relaxing. We went out to dinner and, after a few drinks, the tears came again. I was able to let it all out and talk about it with my mam and sister. It felt good to be able to let my emotions out but even after a good cry and a great weekend I still felt like something was missing. I enjoyed going out to dinner and having a few drinks but I felt that I would have been much happier if I was pregnant and unable to have a few drinks.

I knew what I wanted. I wanted another baby.

Dave's recollections . . .

WHEN I BROUGHT SIOBHÁN HOME after we had lost the baby it was horrible. What could I do? I tried to comfort her. I put my hand on her hand. I put my arm around her shoulder but she pushed me away. Nothing I said or did seemed to get through to her. She was a million miles away from me and I did not know how to get her back. I had cried but she had not. It was like she was trying not to cry. She seemed to be using all her willpower to ignore what was happening.

No matter what I did that day, I kept thinking about the previous night, just before it all happened, when Siobhán and I were lying together in bed and my baby was literally centimetres from me, but now he or she was gone. I kept thinking of the pain Siobhán must have gone through and kept wondering why they wouldn't let me into the emergency room in the hospital. I then started thinking of my own loss. This was my baby, whom I had thought about; I had lots of plans for this little person – if it was a girl I would have done this or if it was a boy I would have done that. All those thoughts meant nothing anymore because there was no baby anymore. It was almost too awful to be true.

I was sitting there in a daze and trying not to cry but at the same time I was aware that Margaret, Siobhán's mam, was sitting beside me, in pain too. Not only had she lost a grandchild, not only was she worried about Siobhán and me, but it must have been bringing back painful memories about the baby she lost, so many years ago. I did not know how to comfort her; I could barely stand thinking about it myself. I was afraid to talk about it; I did not know what to say. Was there anything that would make me feel better? Despite how she must have been feeling too, she did what she always does; she ran around thinking of others. She ran a bath for Siobhán, she cleaned the kitchen, washed the clothes and she made me what seemed like 50 sandwiches and 100 cups of tea that day. I think she was trying to do normal things, to pass the time. I tried to be upbeat but it was awful just sitting there, feeling totally useless. I felt like I was waiting for something to happen but I did not know what.

After she had a few hours' sleep, Siobhán came back downstairs. It was so strange looking at her. She seemed so fragile and so very, very distant. The phone was ringing but she did not want to talk to anyone. The only person she spoke to at all was her sister Sabrina in Jersey. Even that was a quick conversation. Siobhán explained everything and got off the phone very quickly, explaining that she was fine. There were no tears from her. Again, more tears from me. I couldn't help it but she was holding it all in. She is usually so emotional but somehow she held it together. I was a blubbering mess and she was very cool – which is quite the opposite of how we usually are. She is usually so open with her emotions but she never let them out that day – she really bottled it all up.

This was not a day for cooking but still we had to eat. I decided to go to the local Pizza Hut for some dinner; while I was waiting for the food a certain song began to play in the restaurant: "Is it getting better, or do you feel the same?" Instantly I was back in my car outside the hospital. Tears were flowing down my face. One of my wife's sisters decided to come with me and, as she was so young, I didn't want Denise to witness me being so upset, so I kept my back to her. I'm sure she knew I was upset but probably thought it best just to leave me. As I stood there in Pizza Hut, crying my eyes out, the girl behind the counter turned around and, obviously not seeing the tears, asked if I wanted extra cheese on my pizza. I almost laughed at the madness. I was crying my eyes out but had to decide on a pizza topping! Things like that just reminded me that life goes on; the girl was only doing her job and I had to dry my eyes and answer her. I realised that I just had to get a grip; I needed to compose myself, collect our food and get back home. I had a little family to look after; they were depending on me to be strong and I felt I needed to hold it together – at the very least, for them.

The phone rang a lot that night, family and friends passing on their best wishes, asking if there was anything they could do. Siobhán would not take any calls, so I had to take them. More often than not, I was consoling them. I know people were trying to help and it was one of the hardest calls they ever had to make to us. However, when they'd say things like, "Don't worry, you can have more children" or "It just wasn't supposed to be", I have to say, that didn't really help. I think the only thing someone can say is, "I'm thinking of you and if

there's anything I can do . . ." Perhaps the best re-
sponses were from those who offered to make some
dinners, or to call over and take Mitchell out for an
hour's walk – those are the kind of things that definitely helped us!

I was very lucky with work; they gave me a few
days' off so the three of us could be together. The
first few days were very hard. I kept thinking of
Siobhán, about the horrors she had been through,
but then I would think of the baby and every time I
did, I turned from the person who couldn't cry to
this new blubbering idiot. I cried a lot. I was very
surprised how much this tragedy affected me. I was
gutted. What I found the strangest was how quiet
my wife was and how little she wanted to talk
about it. If I was upset Siobhán would comfort me
for a minute or so, and go back to what she was doing. Also, because Mitchell was only ten months
old, he took a lot of our time. We had to play with
him, feed him, clean him and go to the shops to buy
food for him and us.

We seemed to be getting on with things by not
talking about it. I had all these feelings and would
occasionally cry but I don't think I mourned the
baby for the first month. I had so much to say but
no one to listen. I definitely cried a bit but Siobhán
did not want to talk about it, so I did not really
have the chance to say all the things I wanted to
say. I had to keep a lot of my thoughts to myself.
This created a tension at home between Siobhán

and me because we were not dealing with our loss.
We were on different wavelengths. She was in denial and I was trying to be in mourning. It was a
very strange time.

I also found it very hard to communicate with
family and friends because I always felt that they
were uncomfortable talking about the loss. Even
work colleagues, when I returned to work, didn't
really know what to say to me. A couple of them
gathered around me when I returned and asked
about Siobhán but it was clear to me that they only
wanted a quick answer. I said we were sad but that
we would be fine. Once that was said, I could see
that they were visibly relieved that it was talked
about and over with, so they could move on to the
next topic. Apart from the awkwardness of trying
to talk about it, no one seemed to really ask about
me. I felt like all our family and friends concen-
trated on asking after Siobhán, with some male
friends even saying, "Thank God we don't have to
go through it" – but I *was* going through it. I was
confused and frustrated. I had this pain but I
couldn't talk about it. In the first couple of months
only three people (who know who they are) asked
after me *and* Siobhán.

It makes me wonder why so many people think
this just affects women. It also affects the hopes and
dreams of the men who have lost their baby too. I
wish family and friends had been more understanding towards me at that difficult time. I wish

they had wanted to talk to me about it. Unfortunately, not many people wanted to, so I felt that I had to keep it all inside.

A week after we lost the baby, Siobhán decided that she needed "a new project". This "project" was to get a new house. We had been talking about this when Siobhán had still been pregnant but we were only looking on a casual basis. Once we had lost the baby Siobhán threw herself into looking for a new house. She drove me mad. She had me looking through brochure after brochure and scouring the internet for a new house. Looking back on it now I realise this was her way of not dealing with the loss but I did not know how to handle her, so I went along with it. I knew she was jumping into something to keep her mind occupied but what could I do? There was no reasoning with her, she was so angry all the time. I just wanted to make her happy, so I went along with it. I honestly thought it would take us months to find the perfect house so I encouraged her. I thought it might cheer her up to start looking. She was determined to find one and to find it fast and the funny thing about Siobhán is that when she wants something badly, she normally gets it. Personally, I wasn't up for moving as I was still very down about the baby, but she insisted so we kept looking in the newspapers and the internet. Three days later we found the perfect house.

Within a week we had put a deposit down. It all happened so fast. My head was a mess; I didn't know what was going on, I was experiencing the euphoria of purchasing a beautiful new house but still hadn't come to terms with the loss of our baby. We had a new focus now, moving house. We talked a lot about the new house, what we would do with this room and that room and so on. We actually spoke more about the house than the baby until the breakthrough, which came a month after we lost the baby.

It was all thanks to a counsellor at the hospital. When leaving the hospital Siobhán had been advised to see the counsellor to talk about coping with the loss. She did not think she needed to go but after many heated debates, she finally agreed to go along. She seemed to be going just to make me happy. I don't think she was really going for her own sake. I had repeatedly told her how worried I was about her, especially as she was very angry all the time and because she had not been crying; because of that, she made the appointment.

Not long after she left the counsellor, Siobhán was sobbing her heart out. She was trying, through sobs and gushes of tears, to tell me how sad she was, how utterly devastated she was about the baby. That week we mourned together for the first time since we had lost our baby. It was the time the two of us talked, explaining how we both felt and how terrible it was. Most evenings we would talk about it and sometimes I would cry the next day, just thinking about the previous night's conversation. I could be in my car, driving to or from work, and I would start to cry. I was so relieved to be able to talk with Siobhán and it started to bring all sorts of emotions out in me. That week we shared our thoughts and I thought we were really starting to communicate again. I felt we were beginning to understand and be there for each other.

After a week of talking about it, for some reason we stopped talking again. I don't know why but I started to become angry and resentful about losing our baby. I had stopped being upset and had moved on to wondering why it had happened. It was frustrating that there were no answers. It was just something we had to accept and I found it hard to accept. I took these frustrations out on Siobhán. It was unfair really; she had just started coming to terms with the loss and I started getting really angry about it and taking it out on her.

The counsellor had told Siobhán to keep a daily diary, just to write down how she was coping or what she was doing. This proved to be a good avenue for her but I didn't do anything like that and for the next month or two I was finding myself getting angry over little things, taking my frustrations out on Siobhán, shouting and moaning about little things. I have since read my wife's diary and can see that I hurt her, unintentionally of course, but still I hurt her. I hurt her because I was bottling up my feelings. I was angry but I did not want to tell her I was angry. She was learning to cope and grieve and perhaps I did not want to drag her down. I should have just been open with her but I was not. Instead I spent hours on my Playstation, in our study by myself, angrily playing silly games. I was frustrated if I lost a game. I was frustrated if Siobhán asked me to leave the Playstation alone and talk to her. I was frustrated over silly little things. I did not mean to be bad to her but I know I was.

I felt so low and it was at this stage that I realised the only way to move on was with Siobhán, talking together, telling each other how we felt. Communication became very important. We were able to talk again. We were moving on. It was around this time that Siobhán started talking about trying for another baby . . .

Chapter 4

Trying for Another Baby

Siobhán's recollections . . .

MANY PEOPLE HAD BEEN SAYING to me that I was lucky to already have a child, so that at least I could take some comfort in that. That was usually followed by the suggestion that I could always have more children as well. What I had begun to realise was that I had lost a child and that nothing could ever, ever, replace that loss. I lost our baby. I lost my baby. Yes, I had a child already but that is separate from the fact that I had just lost a baby. I don't think it would have mattered if I had one child, two children or three children – I had lost a baby and that, in itself, is a tragedy. That baby was a life that was growing inside me. We had hopes and dreams and plans that involved that baby and now, not only was the baby gone but the vision of our lives, with the baby as part of it, had changed – forever.

Holidays we were planning for the four of us would never happen. Conversations we had about Christmas with two babies were now null and void. All of those hopes and dreams had changed and that was very hard to accept. I know I was very lucky that I had my son at home to cuddle because he always made me feel better but as much as he helped, all the cuddles in the world could not fill the void that had been left. Nothing could take away the pain of the loss I felt for the baby I would never know. It was great to have a little ten-month-old to keep me busy and I was so glad to have him but it did not detract from the emptiness I felt. I felt hollow. No amount of cuddles from my son, shopping trips with my friends, weekends away with my mam or nice dinners with my husband could take away from that.

I guess people were trying to be nice by referring to my son or to the fact that I could have more children. All I could think about was that I might not be able to have any more children. Sure, I had a healthy son at home but I was worried there might be some medical reason for the miscarriage and that it would affect any future pregnancies – should there even be any other pregnancies. I was terrified. I had a friend who had lost a baby and, despite her best efforts, despite hundreds of prayers and positive thoughts from family and friends, she did not conceive again. She went through IVF and a lot of heartache in trying to have a baby but it did not happen for her. Eventually she decided to adopt and now she is a wonderful mother to a gorgeous little boy. The road to becoming a mother was a rocky one for her and it took a long time but she got there eventually and she is very happy now.

I remember speaking with her after we lost the baby. I told her how sad I was and how worried I was that I would never conceive again. She reassured me that there was always a way. Although she had not been able to conceive again, even with IVF, it had all been worth it in the end when she adopted her son. She said as long as I stayed positive, there would be more children in the future for me. It might not be as I had planned it but if I truly wanted it, then it would happen. Her words were so comforting at the time.

As I obsessed about losing my baby, the previous medical problems I had suffered and the fear that I would not be able to get pregnant again, I worried that I might have a similar struggle on my hands on the road to having another baby. I worried if I was up to the kind of a challenge that IVF or adoption can bring. However, I felt in my heart that there were more children in store for us and I knew I would go through IVF, adoption or just about anything to have them. I have colleagues and friends who have bravely gone through it and while it is extremely tough (that's really an understatement because I believe it is a real test of spirit), I felt that I could do it too. If I could not become pregnant again I knew it would devastate me for a while but it would not stop me. It does not stop so many women out there, women who are meant to be mothers but for some reason cannot conceive naturally and I was determined it would not stop me either. I was so sure that Mitchell would have sisters and brothers and I knew I would go through whatever was necessary to make that happen.

So when family or friends were telling me not to worry, that I would be pregnant again in no time, I felt a kind of despair running through me. I know that they did not know what to say to me at that time. I understand that they were just trying to say the right thing, to try to make me feel better, but I used to get a little shiver down my spine at the mention of becoming pregnant again – that shiver was the fear that I would not. I did not share those feelings with the well-wishers; it would not have done anybody any good. I only shared those desperate thoughts with my husband.

Even if they were not saying what I wanted to hear, I do appreciate the people who called to the house or picked up the phone, for having the courage to come and see me or just talk to me. I know it was hard for them too, especially as they thought they were saying the right things by reminding me how lucky I was to have Mitchell at home and assuring me I would pregnant again very soon.

What I felt like saying is that having a child already or becoming pregnant again are wonderful things but they are separate from the baby we lost and are not compensation for that loss. It is wonderful to be a mother but it would not be fair to make Mitchell compensate me for the child I had lost. Also, I knew (somewhere in the back of my mind) that it would not be right to try to become pregnant to replace the baby that had been lost; still, that's exactly what I wanted to do.

I wanted to be pregnant immediately. I wanted to start trying as soon as humanly possible. We lost our baby on February 25th and I wanted to be pregnant by April. Unfortunately, I was not feeling very sexual or attractive after what I had been through, so I was not exactly in the mood for romancing my husband, but I definitely wanted to get pregnant as soon as I could. I thought that becoming pregnant again would fill the empty feeling I had been experiencing since our baby had gone away. I know it's wrong to say that a pregnancy could fill the void, but as I am trying to be *completely honest* here, and even though I knew I could never replace the baby I lost, I thought being pregnant would make the emptiness go away.

And so, I was on a mission to get pregnant. I just had to figure out the best way to get pregnant as quickly as possible. I had suffered from heavy bleeding for quite a few days after the miscarriage. Then again, two weeks after that, I had suffered from more bleeding. I thought it best to get a regular menstrual cycle back before trying to become pregnant again. As much as I wanted to be pregnant right away, I waited for a few weeks until I thought it was safe to start trying again. They were the longest weeks of my life. I was so impatient. I wanted to be pregnant but I knew I should wait. I was also still worried sick that I would not be able to get pregnant. I was scared that something might be wrong with me and that I would never have another baby. I became totally obsessed; it consumed my thoughts. At that time, thoughts of another baby was the antidote to my grief.

By the end of March everything settled down with my menstrual cycle and I wanted to start trying. My husband was a little apprehensive but I was so determined that he eventually (even reluctantly) agreed. I think he was secretly hoping it would not happen but he gave in to me because I was very, very convincing. I tried to convince him that I was fine; besides, I reminded him that I had been to the counsellor and with the homework she had given me of writing into my diary every night, I was able to vent my emotions through that and I felt that I was almost back to being myself. So I said, trying my very best to convince him (or maybe I was trying to convince myself) that it was not an attempt to have a replacement baby. I simply said that we had always wanted more children and we wanted to have them close together, so it made sense to start trying immediately.

Someone up there must have agreed with him because in April we tried but it did not happen. I thought I was pregnant at first. My period was about four days late and I have always been pretty regular, so I was expecting to be pregnant. I went out and bought a pregnancy test and when I took it the results were "inconclusive". There was a bit of blurring on it but it was not at all clear. I went crazy over that test result. I stared at it for hours, trying to see if it was or was not positive.

I kept staring at it until my husband came in from work and then I made him examine it. I was losing my mind again. He reckoned it was negative and after he threw it in the bin, he sat me down and asked me to be patient. He pleaded with me to wait and see what happened over the next few days. I meekly agreed and told him that I would be patient and that he shouldn't worry about me. The test was in the bin and I promised him I would not take any more tests. I would just wait to see whether my period would arrive or not. To him I'm sure I seemed calm. So when he left me sitting at the kitchen table, he probably thought he had gotten through to me, he probably thought I would wait . . .

I was never known for my great patience and as soon as he was gone out of the room, I had the test out of the bin and was back to examining it again. I was definitely losing the plot. I had myself convinced that I was pregnant. I thought my boobs were tender. I thought my tummy was a bit icky. I thought my sense of smell was heightened.

I was obviously imagining these symptoms because, the very next day, my period arrived. I was devastated – again. I had been so sure that I was pregnant and once I discovered that I was not, I was so upset. It was like another loss. It felt like a failed attempt to me. I cried my eyes out when my period arrived that morning and I was still sobbing regularly that evening, when Dave came home from work. He was very reassuring that it would happen when the time was right. He suggested that perhaps my body was just not ready yet. After all, (God bless him for trying to reason with me) he reminded me, it had only been two months since we had lost the baby and I was still not back into a proper menstrual cycle yet. My body needed time to heal before I could embark on another pregnancy – and so did my mind. I needed enough time for my hormones to balance themselves out before I could become pregnant again. I can assure you, my hormones were definitely not back to normal at that stage because I was raging, devastated and totally frustrated that day. Another month had gone by and another period had arrived. I was sad and angry all over again. I felt like I had missed a chance to become pregnant. It sounds crazy saying it like that now but that's how I felt.

Dave said all the right things but it did not help me one little bit. He was supportive, loving, understanding and reassuring. But not one word of what he said, even though he was absolutely right (its not often I admit that), got through to me. In my mind it was another failure. I had tried to conceive and I had failed – again. There was no reasoning with me. Perhaps it was my hormones making me crazy or perhaps it was because I was a mother who had lost her baby and needed so badly to fill the void that my only mission in life was to become pregnant again and every failed attempt was a horrific reminder of the emptiness that enveloped me since I had lost my baby. I could not stand it. It was overwhelming. It was all I could think about.

Suddenly I was very jealous of every pregnant woman I saw. I would take my son out most days for a walk or to the park or playgroup and it seemed I would run into more women who were pregnant than those who were not. I did not even live anywhere near a maternity hospital but there seemed to be pregnant women all around me. I don't know where they all came from. Perhaps they were there before but at that time, it was as if my senses had been heightened and I was acutely aware of any bumps around me.

I was so jealous. Everywhere I looked there were happy pregnant people, rubbing their baby bumps lovingly, and I was feeling very *not* pregnant. It was such a hard time for me. I remember often gazing at pregnant bellies as they walked past me and sometimes I would unconsciously rub my own empty tummy. Then I would look down at my non-pregnant belly and I would get very, very upset. I felt so hollow. It was an awful feeling.

A good friend of mine, Lynn, was pregnant at that time and I was afraid to see her in case I would become upset or jealous by the sight of her being heavily pregnant. I remember she phoned me up to say she was planning to call over to my house for lunch. I appreciated the courage it must have taken for her to phone me and so I did not want to ask her not to come over for lunch. I decided I would just have to face her and hope for the best. I knew it was awkward for her even to call me. Even though a part of me wanted to ask her not to come, I knew I needed to get over that fear and see her.

I was very apprehensive as I made the soup and sandwiches. I had a knot in my stomach when the doorbell rang. However, when she came in with her lovely big pregnant belly, she looked so radiant and happy I could not help but be genuinely happy for her. It was such a relief; I was not at all uneasy around her. We had a lovely lunch and a good chat and I felt so much better after it. I will always be grateful to her for having the courage to come to see me. She was so brave to come over while she was pregnant, knowing I was very sad about not being pregnant anymore. Thanks for that, Lynn; it meant the world to me.

So I was on a mission. I wanted to get pregnant. I decided it was not the most romantic time in our lives and telling my husband that we had to "do it" on days 11, 12, 13 and 14 was not the ideal way for it to happen. Besides, I wanted our baby to be conceived naturally, in love – not military style – so I suggested we go out and have a nice romantic meal (on day 12, but that's beside the point).

My husband left Mitchell to his nana's house so they could have him for the night, while I stayed at home and got ready. I had been feeling really dowdy since I had lost the baby and I had not been making much of an effort to look nice (how could I think about make up when I felt like crying all the time?) but I wanted to look good that night, so I decided to make a real effort. I went out and bought a new outfit and got my hair done. I spent ages doing make-up and nails and I felt completely transformed by the time I was finished getting ready.

By the time he got home, I was dressed and ready to go. He nearly had a heart attack at the sight of me. Either he was genuinely happy and in love with his good-looking wife or he's one hell of an actor! Although, in fairness, I had been an awful sight for two months and he was probably genuinely delighted (or relieved?) that I was starting to look like "me" again.

I was chuffed to be all dressed up and going out as we left the house. It had been a long time since we had gone out and I wanted to make the most of it. We had a drink before dinner and then headed into the restaurant. We ordered some wine and a lovely meal and we chatted about all sorts of things. It was such a wonderful, romantic evening. We had great fun . . . until we started to talk about the baby. As the dessert arrived, the two of us had teary eyes and we were struggling to hold back the tears. I couldn't help it; I started to cry first. I could not help thinking that I would have been five months pregnant at that time, if the baby had not been lost. We sat there and cried over our ice cream. After a while, the waiter brought us our bill and tried not to look too closely at the woman with mascara running down her cheeks and the man with the red eyes. He dropped the bill and practically sprinted away from the table.

We went home, cuddled up in bed, cried a little bit more, laughed about the waiter running a mile at the look of us and then we made love. After all, we were in love and although we were still sad, we had enjoyed a beautiful evening together and we decided it would not be at all bad if a baby was conceived that night.

Two weeks later I was anticipating the tender boobs, increased awareness to smells and mood swings. All that came was the mood swings. Some people would say that "one out of three isn't bad", but not my husband. If you lived with me, you would understand. I can sometimes get a little bit cranky (that might be a bit of an understatement) when my period is due to arrive. For a few days coming up to it I can be "out of sorts", to say the least, and this month was worse than usual. I was like a woman possessed.

Again, I imagined all the symptoms. I thought I had the nose of a bloodhound; I thought my boobs were tender. I thought I was extra tired and starting to feel a little bit nauseous. I thought I was going to be taking a test and that it would be positive. I was so sure it had happened this time. I was on the verge of getting excited when . . . yep, you've guessed it, my period arrived.

I was completely devastated – again. I was getting really worried that I might never get pregnant again. My mind kept going back to my early twenties, when I had suffered serious health problems, which had affected my fertility. I thought these problems were coming back and the idea of that terrified me. I imagined all sorts of things going on inside my body. I was sure I would never have any more children. I could not see the positive side . . .

I remembered the horror of what I had gone through some years earlier and I prayed I would not have to go through that again. I had suffered from ovarian cysts for seven years. It was a nightmare. Apart from all the pain, there was the worry about the damage the cysts could have been doing to my fertility; I ended up on the operating table more than once to try to sort out the problem. It was a long time before it was resolved.

After three failed attempts at keyhole surgery, I eventually had to undergo a Caesarean section-style operation because they were unable to remove the cyst through keyhole surgery. That time when they opened me up, they found a cyst the size of a grapefruit. It was entangled around my left ovary and part of my fallopian tube. They had to untangle it to remove it. Along with the cyst, they ended up removing part of my left ovary where it had been damaged. They tried their best to repair the damage but it was not all good news. When I woke up, I was in so much pain, but what the doctor told me was worse than all the pain in the world. He explained what had happened during the operation and, while he said it had been "successful" in removing the cyst completely, he also explained that I might have problems when trying to conceive.

I had been left with one ovary, a partially damaged fallopian tube and the worry that I might never have children. It was not hopeless but the surgeon said it might be "difficult". That was an awful thing to find out nine months before I was due to get married. Dave and I really wanted to have children and I was terrified I would not be able to. Over the next few months the doctors kept an eye on me and the cyst did not return. I felt good and healthy and was free from pain, so I just hoped that I would be able to have children one day. I tried not to dwell on the negative and instead saw myself being a mammy one day.

You can imagine my surprise when I discovered I had become pregnant on our honeymoon! We had said we would go with the flow and not use any contraception once we got married and we would just wait and see what happened. Our son, Mitchell, is what happened. By the time we were on our flight home I was peeing every five minutes. By the time we got back home I was feeling a bit strange. A few days later I had tender boobs, my sense of smell was heightened and I was peeing on to a stick. We were delighted to discover I was pregnant.

Two years later, having had a baby and lost a baby, I was desperately trying to get pregnant again. But because my period had arrived again, I was afraid that perhaps something had gone wrong when I lost the baby. I thought something inside me got damaged and I was terrified I would never get pregnant again. I wondered about the medical instruments they had used to help me deliver the baby: did they cause me some internal damage that I did not know about? Should they have given me a D&C anyway? I was afraid that a part of the placenta could have been left inside and that maybe it had gone bad and caused me irreparable damage?

I was losing the plot but I could not help it. My mind was again consumed with fears that I would never have another baby. I knew I had been lucky to get pregnant in the first place almost two years earlier. I knew I was extremely lucky that I had a problem-free pregnancy, which resulted in my gorgeous little boy. I knew I was very lucky to get pregnant a second time around, even if it was a little sooner than we had anticipated. So when we lost that baby and I was unable to get pregnant after three months of trying, I had started to panic. I should not even say that I was "unable to get pregnant", because three months of trying is hardly a failure, especially when you consider that some people spend years trying. However, to me, at that time and because of how empty I felt inside, three months felt like an eternity.

So my period had arrived and I was definitely not pregnant – again. I was so upset. As the counsellor had recommended, I had kept a diary since my first visit with her. I had got into the habit of writing into my diary every night and that night's entry went as follows:

21st May

Definitely not pregnant – I got my period today. I was hoping so much that I might be pregnant, but no luck. I have kept myself busy this week trying not to think about it but it's at the forefront of my thoughts. I am so devastated that my period came today. It was horrible. It was so painful and heavy. I kept going all day to get through it and take my mind off it but I still feel completely empty inside. I should be 24 weeks' pregnant now. The only thing that can take away this empty feeling is to be pregnant again. I am going to pray that it happens next month. I don't want to face another period. I don't think I can take the heartache. I miss my baby so much. It's so unfair. I have so much love to give and I desperately want more children to give it to. I'll always have a special love for the baby we lost but I also want to move on and have another little baby. I want to feel a new life grow inside me.

Dave's recollections . . .

When we lost the baby I felt then, as I do now (this is me being scientific), that Siobhán's body was not ready to grow a new baby so quickly after having our first boy. He was only seven months old when she got pregnant again and I believe it was nature saying "no, not yet, she's just not ready".

After we began talking about the loss and moving on a bit, Siobhán decided she wanted to be pregnant again. I didn't share that opinion at the time. I felt she wasn't ready physically or mentally and, to be honest, I don't think I was mentally ready either. However, such is married life that I was told to be ready at certain times in the month and I did what I was told. Even though I was not convinced it was the right way to go about it I wanted more children too and another baby would be wonderful. So I did what I was asked to do on days 11, 12, 13 and 14. After all, my job wasn't that hard, was it?

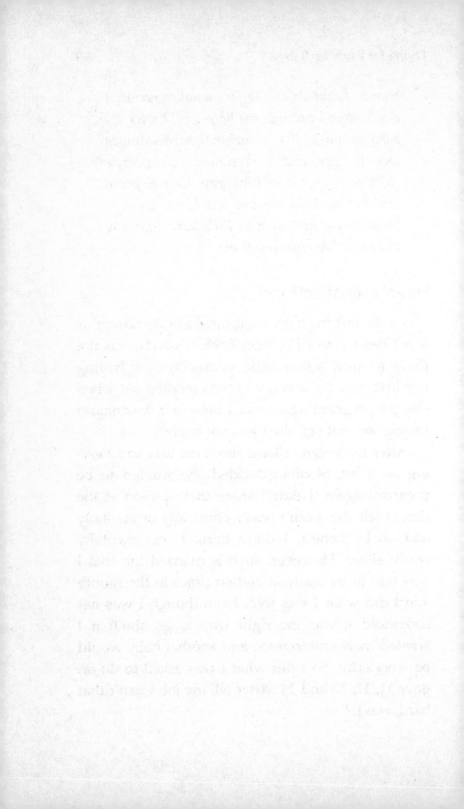

Chapter 5

Getting on with Life

Siobhán's recollections . . .

I WAS DUE BACK TO THE COUNSELLOR that week. I did not have anyone to look after the little man, so I took him with me. He is a very good little boy and he played on the floor happily while I chatted with the counsellor. I talked about my need to get pregnant again. I told her how I was very frustrated and not happy because it was not happening. She suggested that if I was a bit more relaxed about it, then perhaps it would happen naturally. We talked for an hour and I felt good afterwards. I was dealing with the loss of the baby quite well, so we decided that I did not need to go back to her again, unless, of course, I felt like I needed to at some time in the future. However, at that point, I felt like I was dealing with everything OK. I was feeling pretty optimistic and confident about the future.

Just before I left, she asked me if my baby had been a boy or a girl. I was surprised by this question. I had told her my story about how I had lost and indeed never seen the baby but she was asking me this question, to which I did not have the answer. She said I should decide if it was a boy or a girl. She said it was important for me to make up my mind about that. I said I would think about it but honestly, I was confused about why she was asking me to do this. I did not challenge her about it at the time because in my mind she was the counsellor and supposedly knew best. I just wanted to do what she asked me to, especially if I thought it would make me feel better. However, since that day I've spent a lot of time thinking about whether my baby was a boy or a girl and to be honest I have never come to a decision. Looking back, I think she was wrong to ask me that question. I don't understand why she told me it was so important to decide this and I don't think she should have put extra pressure on me in this way. I have no way of knowing and I feel it was unfair and unprofessional of her to ask me to decide this.

Aside from her asking me about the sex of the baby and interrupting me every so often to tell me things about herself and her own family, I did have a positive experience with her and, as I left, I promised her that I would continue to write into my diary each night, as this was proving an excellent way of venting my emotions without killing anyone (namely Dave).

Despite feeling disappointed about not being pregnant, my mind was occupied with other things. We had decided to move house, so I was being kept busy with that. We had lots of viewings of our own house, which we were trying to sell, so I was kept on my toes preparing it for these viewings. After a few weeks, when we were still waiting for the right offer, I had started to feel stressed again. I felt like my dream house was slipping away from me because, if we could not sell our house, then we could not move. Finally, after what seemed like an age, we got the offer we wanted for our house. We then had to get ready for the move to the new house. It was a busy time and I was very excited about the move. We were buying a house by the seaside and I could not wait to get back to living by the sea with the lovely fresh sea air. We had our lives back on track and we were focusing on the future and not dwelling on the past. Things were looking up. Moving house, although it was a hectic and stressful time, was a very positive thing for me because it totally distracted me from the feelings of sadness that had been consuming me. It gave me a project to throw myself into. I guess sometimes a distraction is good therapy to a loss, as it was giving me so much to look forward to.

I had stopped obsessing about becoming pregnant. I had stopped being a crazy person. I had come to realise that if I continued to panic about not getting pregnant then it would never happen. I knew that I needed to be calm and relaxed and that it would happen when the time was right and, if it did not happen, then we would look into other available options. The main thing that was important for me was that I was no longer feeling hopeless or like a failure just because I was not pregnant. I had decided that a baby may or may not come our way naturally. If it did, wonderful; and if it did not, well, that would be a bridge we would cross if and when the time came. I felt calm and hopeful. I felt like I could deal with either outcome. I was beginning to feel good about myself and our future again.

One of my diary entries from that week went as follows:

15th June

Everything is going great at the moment. The move is coming up soon and I can't wait. Our house is in the process of being sold and everything is falling into place. I am so excited about it. I cleaned the house for hours today and that is usually a sign that my period is on the way. I am not sure if it is, we'll just have to wait and see. I am not taking any tests this time; I am just going to wait. I thought about our baby a lot today. I know I'll never stop being sad about our baby but hopefully we'll have more children in the future and that will help. Mitchell is a great help, he keeps me so distracted. He is so clever and funny and I love him so much. He takes some of the pain away because he is so wonderful and he keeps me so busy but I know the pain will never be gone completely and I guess it should not be. I need to have a little bit of sadness to stay close to my baby and I suppose I need to find a way to live with that.

It was good for our marriage (and my sanity) that I had decided to stop fretting about getting pregnant and just let things happen their own way, in their own time. Around that time (possibly because I was no longer a ticking time-bomb) Dave decided to take a week off work, so we could spend some proper time together. We wanted to unwind and relax for a few days before the house move, so we decided to head out of Dublin for some fresh country air. We had got married in Glendalough in Wicklow, so we decided to go down there for a day. The three of us headed off. It was a gorgeous day as we walked around the Lough. Afterwards, we went into the hotel for lunch. It should have been a happy and romantic day; after all we were surrounded by beautiful countryside and we were having lunch in the hotel where our wedding reception had been held – but things did not go quite as we had planned.

I don't know if it was my fault or his but we
ended up having a huge argument in the car as we
left the hotel. We had not been getting on well that
day and it all came to a head as we left. I demanded
he stop the car (in the middle of the countryside)
and let me out. I hopped out, closed the door and
walked off. In keeping with the madness, he drove
off. I sat there in the lovely June sunshine and just
contemplated things. After a few minutes I could
not even remember what had started the argument.
I was actually feeling pretty calm and peaceful
when he drove back to get me a few minutes later.
He pulled up beside me and sat there in the car. I
sat there on the side of the road. It was so silly. I
don't even know why we were fighting or whose
fault it was, but he would not get out of the car to
say sorry and I would not get into the car to say
sorry. Mitchell was asleep in the back of the car, so
he was oblivious to the craziness.

As I sat there on the wall, trying my best to be
defiant and angry, I eventually burst out laughing
(if ever someone should have come to take me
away in a white coat, it was at that moment) and as
I looked over to him, he was sitting in the car, trying his best not to laugh. I got into the car and we
both laughed. It was so silly. It was all over nothing. I think sometimes we all need to blow off a little steam and unfortunately, it's those nearest and
dearest to us who bear the brunt of it.

We went home and managed to have a lovely evening. We talked about the baby a lot that week. We talked about how far gone in the pregnancy I would have been. We talked about how the hospital should change their policy and allow husbands or partners in the emergency room for situations like that. (I will never understand that policy. I complained to the counsellor about it but no one ever followed up with me about why that is the hospital policy.) We talked about the sadness that we still felt every day. We talked about how our hearts had been broken but were slowly mending, although we suspected that there would always be a little crack left from all the sadness we had been through. We were at a place where we could have open conversations about it and although there were still some tears shed, we had come to accept what had happened and we were dealing with it. We talked, excitedly, about the upcoming move to the new house. Overall, life was good. We were healthy, happy and excited about our future.

I was also no longer completely obsessed about becoming pregnant. I resigned myself to the thought that I would have to have faith and believe that we would have more children in the future. I felt it in my heart and I just knew that it would happen for us when the time was right.

We had a few romantic evenings that week, so it could have been any one of them. I'm not quite sure when the magic happened but two weeks and two

blue lines later, I was thrilled. We were truly delighted to discover that I was pregnant. We were
both over the moon. We had our lives back on
track. Mitchell was doing great, walking and talking and getting up to all kinds of mischief. We were
about to move into a lovely new house. It was perfect timing for our new baby to be on the way.

17th July

*I am trying not to get my hopes up, I really am.
But today I thought my period came and I
almost had a heart attack. I really think the
blood drained from my face. I was in total shock
and despair until I ran to the bathroom and
discovered that it was not my period. I am three
days late and the test was positive – it was faint
but it was definitely positive. It will be so great
if I am pregnant but I am trying so hard (and
failing miserably) not to put all my hopes on it
because my period could arrive tomorrow . . .*

Those were a tense few days. I had all the feelings
of a pregnant woman but I was so excited that I
might be that I tried my best not to pin all my hopes
on it. I could not wipe the smile off my face one
minute and the next I was fretting about the possibility that my period could arrive at any minute.
The positive result was so wonderful and I was delighted but I was so nervous and apprehensive that

I wanted to wait until I was more certain before taking any more tests.

22ⁿᵈ July

Definitely pregnant!!! I took another test today and it was positive – very positive!! The line was very blue. I am thrilled. I feel so content. I was a bit emotional today (so what's new). I felt like I wanted to cry one minute, kill someone the next minute and hug someone the minute after that. . . so I stayed away from people all day. I am so delighted but I am not forgetting about our lost baby. On September 11ᵗʰ we will have a special day, dedicated to our baby who would have been due that day. We might plant a tree in the garden of our new house if we have moved in by then. I would love to plant a tree in memory of our baby on that special day. It means I will have somewhere special to go to talk to the baby – our little angel who might be gone but is still looking over us somehow.

Dave's recollections . . .

At first when we started trying for another baby, I felt that we were not ready. I felt like there was something missing. Maybe I felt it was too soon because I knew we hadn't gotten over the baby we had lost, but then I realised I'd probably never get over such a sad event and maybe a new baby could not only help us feel better but that it might bring us together as a family. One or two of the months we got quite close; in fact I believe in month two (of trying) that Siobhán got pregnant again but it failed to materialise after the first week.

During this time we were more open in our discussions about the baby. It's funny (and I'm still the same) but whenever we spoke about the baby I would be fine that day but I would always burst into tears the following day.

About three months after we had lost our baby, the two of us were in a much better place. We were happier together and progressing well with our grief. We were relaxed and open with each other and we (or should I say, Siobhán) were no longer trying like mad to get pregnant. We had decided to let nature takes its course. This took some pressure off me and I really felt happy about trying, albeit casually, for another baby.

It was around this time Siobhán got pregnant again. I believe it happened because we were back to normal. We had nights where we just relaxed together and we had nights where we drove each other crazy. Like most couples we had times when we fought over nothing, we had times when we laughed over silly things. We were a husband and wife again and we were back to being able to make love very freely (without calculating dates or checking temperatures!). The smiles that had been missing for a few months had found their way back on to our faces and we were happy again. It was the right time for a baby to be conceived and I am glad it did not happen until then because I know our baby girl was conceived in love and not as a replacement for a baby we lost.

Chapter 6

A New Life

Siobhán's recollections . . .

I WAS STILL WRITING INTO MY DIARY when I became pregnant again. I was busy writing into my diary the night I first saw the two blue lines. I was so excited as I scribbled my entry as fast as I could possibly write that it is barely legible to me now. As the days went by and the baby grew stronger I wrote into my diary each night. I wrote down my hopes and fears. I had apprehensions about losing this baby, too. I was terrified I would wake up one day and see blood. I was comforted that I felt so sick (the awful but strangely comforting morning, noon and night sickness) for the first sixteen weeks because I had been very sick with Mitchell for the first thirteen weeks and he had been perfectly healthy when he made his entrance to this world. I had not had any sickness on the baby we had lost, so I was taking the intense nausea with the new baby as a very positive sign. Still, I was very nervous and so we decided that we would not tell anyone about me being pregnant. We wanted to pass the three-month mark before sharing our good news.

It was difficult to keep it quiet because I was feeling very ill but I kept a low profile and did not spend too much time with people for those first few months, so they would not be suspicious. I did not want to tell family and friends in case we lost this baby too, because I did not want to go through the ordeal of having to tell sad news to people again, if the worst came to the worst. It was the first time in my life I was determined to keep something a complete secret. Anyway, I wrote into my diary every night, so that in itself was almost like telling a friend what I was going through.

Life is funny. You can plan things but you cannot control anything. I planned not to tell anyone about my pregnancy but I had no control over my eleven-year-old sister, Kate, who went upstairs to my bedroom and read my diary while I was downstairs in the kitchen making dinner. I had no idea I had left it on top of my dresser. I had no idea she would pick it up and open it and read it all the way to the entry from the night before, which talked about how I was seven weeks pregnant. I had no idea she would continue to read as it went on to say how nervous, apprehensive and excited I was to be going for an early pregnancy ultrasound scan the very next afternoon. I probably should have kept my diary locked away but I forgot to put it away. Kate probably should not have read it, but she was only a child who found a pretty pink book and peeked inside to see what it was.

When she came down the stairs she looked at me differently. She would not quite meet my eyes and so I knew she was up to something. I went upstairs and (I kid you not) she had left the diary open, in the middle of my bed, on the page where I had written the previous night's entry. She knew I was pregnant. I was sure of it. I went back downstairs to speak with her and as I walked into the sitting room, I could hear her telling my thirteen-year-old sister Denise that I was definitely pregnant. I guess they thought I would be mad at them for finding out but I was not. I explained to them that I was nervous because of what had happened last time and that I was planning to tell the family after the early pregnancy scan – once I knew everything was OK.

It turned out they suspected I was pregnant because I had been sucking on liquorice like crazy over the previous weeks, just like I did when I was pregnant with Mitchell! They had been snooping around trying to find out if I was or not and my diary presented them with all the answers they needed, so Kate decided to read the whole thing and find out for sure. Then once she had the information she needed, she shared it all with Denise. Cheeky little monkeys!

The next day we went to the hospital for the scan. We had had so many ups and downs in this hospital. Mitchell had been born there. Our baby had been lost there and now we were to find out about this new little baby. We could only hope the news would be good and that we would be leaving with smiles on our faces. I took my sisters with me because they had stayed with me overnight and I was not letting them out of my sight until I was ready to reveal our secret. I suspected they would spill the beans to my parents, given half a chance. If the news was good, I would tell my family the good news myself. My sisters stayed out in the waiting area and played with Mitchell, as Dave and I went in to find out about the new life growing inside me. I was sick with worry. I was also sick with morning sickness but it was mostly the worry that had my stomach in terrible knots. It was one of the tensest moments of my life.

I must tell you that during my first pregnancy I was very bashful at my hospital appointments. I would only undress if I was specifically asked to do so. I was not keen on revealing too much of my body unless it was absolutely necessary. Going through labour and birth eradicated most of that bashfulness, so by the time I went in for this scan, I was not one bit bothered about stripping off. As I walked over to the bed, I promptly took off my trousers and I was about to take off my knickers when the nurse advised me that I did not need to undress. She looked at me like I was mad as I tried hurriedly to re-dress myself. Oh, the embarrassment of it!

As I tugged at the zip on my trousers, Dave explained to her that we had recently lost a baby and, as such, were very nervous about finding out how this new little baby was coming along. Once we explained that, she was very understanding and sensitive. I could hear Dave talking to her but I think I was in a daze. I was just so nervous that I did not know what I was doing. Dave managed a bit of a laugh with the nurse over my stripping antics but he was also very nervous and she picked up on this and got me set up for the scan as quickly as she could. I'm sure she could tell from our desperately worried expressions, that we just wanted to see our baby on the screen and find out if everything was OK as soon as possible.

Within a few minutes I was semi-undressed and lying up on the bed. My belly was covered with the cold gel and the nurse was pressing into my bladder to get a good view of the baby. As much as my bladder was crying out to be emptied, all my energy went into searching the screen for my baby. Where was she? Was she the right size? Was there a heartbeat? Was it strong? All these questions were buzzing around my head . . . and then I saw her.

It was one of the best moments of my life. There she was, only seven weeks old and already thriving. Her heartbeat was strong and she was moving around like a jumping jellybean. It was incredible. I started to cry, tears of relief and joy. I looked at Dave and he had tears in his eyes too. It was such a special moment – even if it was short-lived, because the need to pee took over and I jumped off the bed and ran (half-dressed) into the bathroom next door. When I came back, the nurse who had been wonderfully sensitive to our situation had kept the picture of our baby up on the screen, so we could look at her for a few minutes when I came back. She told us not to worry, that everything looked great. Our little baby girl was exactly the right size and her heartbeat was healthy and strong. She thanked me for giving her a laugh with my strip-show and then she gave us a little picture of the scan to take home. We walked out of that hospital with the biggest smiles possible on our faces.

We already had our wonderful little boy and now we had confirmation that our new little baby looked perfect. We could not have been happier. It was great telling our families but we kept the news to just family and the odd close friend, until we passed the three-month mark – just in case something did go wrong. Even though we knew from the look of her bouncing around on the screen that she was very strong, we decided to keep it "hush-hush" for a while anyway.

Dave's recollections . . .

WHEN SIOBHÁN SHOWED ME THOSE two first two blues lines which were a little weak and then two strong blue lines a few days later, I was so excited but nervous at the same time. I did not want to get my hopes up and I also wanted to keep it a complete secret. That proved to be quite a struggle for Siobhán, even though she did agree with me that we should keep it to ourselves – well, she agreed at the beginning of the pregnancy anyway. As her morning sickness got worse she complained to me that she found it difficult to keep the news to herself. She drove me mad trying to convince me that we should tell our parents and siblings (as much as she may deny it now) but I pleaded with her to keep it quiet for a bit longer, at least until we had the scan to see how the baby was progressing. She actually managed to keep it under wraps until her sister read her diary and found out about the baby. Try as she might, she was visibly delighted that Kate read her diary. That was the break she needed. That was the licence to tell all and as soon as we had our scan picture, the very next day, she made me drive her straight to both our parents' houses to tell them our good news!

I was excited and hopeful about the pregnancy and our future. Siobhán was very sick and I took this as a good sign because she had been sick on Mitchell but not with the baby we lost. The more she was sick, the more reassured I felt. Although I did feel bad for her, I was relieved to see that the baby had a good strong hold on her already.

Chapter 7

Never Forget

Siobhán's recollections . . .

BEING PREGNANT AGAIN WAS COMPLETELY wonderful. I was delighted (if you can believe it) to have morning sickness for sixteen weeks. The baby had completely taken over my body and mind. I was exhausted and throwing up constantly but I was happy to be that way. There was barely an hour that went by where I did not throw up or feel the urge to throw up but I barely complained (not so sure Dave would agree on that one) about spending most of my time in the bathroom, I was just so happy that the baby was growing well and was so strong. It was a relief in my mind, even if it was a burden on my body.

I must admit that the void I felt, the void that I was so desperate to fill, the void I was so sure I could fill, was *never* filled. It is right that it has never been filled. I know now that it is not possible to fill such a void. It is a part of who I have become and I cherish it now. I was extremely happy to be pregnant with Robyn but, once I was, I realised that the little baby I had growing inside me was not a replacement for a baby I had lost. I would always grieve the loss of our baby and nothing would ever change that. *Nothing should ever change that.* The baby we lost was a dropped stitch in life's tapestry and is part of who we have become. While we would go on with our lives and have more children, what I had finally learned was that this little baby should not be forgotten or replaced. It could not be.

On the day the baby we lost would have been due to be born, we had a very special day in honour of the baby. Dave and I went to a church where we lit a candle and said some prayers for our little lost angel. Then we went to dinner and spent the evening reminiscing about the events that had unfolded. We dedicated that day to remembering the baby we had lost. It was sad, but it was also nice. It was good to set aside some special time just to remember the baby.

I know that on February 25th (the day we lost the baby) and September 11th (the day the baby would have been due) every year for the rest of our lives, we will put some special time aside for the baby because he or she deserves that, at the very least. We also remind family that we will be having a difficult time on those two dates. We don't expect everyone to remember those dates, even though they are ingrained in our heads, so we gently let them know that, if we seem a little bit preoccupied, it's because our minds are drifting to thoughts of the baby we lost. We usually get a positive response from family and friends when we remind them about it and they often tell us they will say a prayer or light a candle in memory of the baby. It's nice to think that those close to us take some time to think about this little life too. It's comforting to us.

We include our children in the remembrance too. We tell them that they had a little baby brother or sister who did not make it into this world but instead was called up to heaven. They are still very young but our son is starting to understand. The baby's anniversary has recently passed and he asked me if the baby is happy up in heaven. I assured him that the baby is very happy. Then he asked me if the baby is playing with Granddad Paddy, who recently passed away, and I answered that he was. "Are they playing football, Mammy?" he wanted to know. Once I assured him that they were playing happily together, Granddad Paddy rolling the ball to the baby with his walking stick, exactly as he used to do with Mitchell and Robyn, he was very contented and went back to his jigsaw. I will always include them in the remembrance so that, hopefully, when they grow up, they will be able to include us in the important things that are going on in their lives too.

But life must go on; we had a new baby coming into the world and we had to be strong and stay positive for her. Once we knew she was growing normally and that everything looked OK, we started to relax and enjoy the pregnancy. As with most pregnancies, we had our good days and our not-so-good days but overall, we were so excited and hopeful about the future. It was like we had been given another chance and we cherished her, even before she was born. It was so wonderful when she finally made an appearance. Our beautiful baby girl, Robyn, arrived four days before her due date and weighed in at a healthy 7lbs ½oz. She is clever, beautiful, wonderful and challenging at times but I am thankful every day for her and her brother. They are my little miracles and while I still think sometimes about what might have been if the baby had made it, I am so very grateful for my family and I love every day I have with them.

Dave's recollections . . .

IT WAS GREAT THAT SIOBHÁN WAS pregnant again, but we never stopped thinking or talking about our lost baby. On the baby's due date we had a very emotionally moving day. It was very hard for me. I wanted to grieve for the baby but I wanted to keep Siobhán calm. She was four months pregnant at this stage and I kept thinking, "Don't let her get upset as this may cause some sadness to our new little one", but with her constant running to the toilet to puke or pee, I felt reassured.

That night, as we were having dinner in one of our favourite restaurants, I felt the tears coming again. I couldn't stop them and, wouldn't you know it, I had yet another big cry, but I didn't care; I was only showing my feelings for my baby. The baby deserves to be remembered, particularly on those special days and I suspect I will shed many tears on those two dates over the coming years, for our little baby who never quite made it.

Of course it is vital to get on with life but it's also important to remember the things that mean most to us. Every year in February and September we will remember.

What helped me through this extraordinarily hard event was Siobhán; the most important thing was to talk about it. Although there were some very hard times, we stuck together, listened to each other and helped each other move forward. In fact, the only times it was really bad was when we did not talk to each other. The times when we did not communicate were the hardest. Losing a baby can really put a strain on a person and it can also be hurtful to a relationship if the couple cannot find a way to be open about their feelings.

We had a tough couple of months at the start. First Siobhán could not cry about it, while I was crying all the time, and then when she finally started to grieve I was at the angry stage and was not talking to her. Luckily for us, we were able to sort ourselves out. Once we stuck together and were there for each other, it all changed. I think it actually made us stronger as a couple. I can definitely understand how couples can break up after such a loss but I can only recommend being honest and open with each other and you'll be able to find a way through it. It still hurts thinking about it now and as I type here, there is a tear in my eye. However, I know I am lucky to have such a strong bond with Siobhán and also, very fortunately for us, we have two amazingly beautiful children to keep us busy here and we know we have a little angel looking after the four of us from above.

Chapter 8

Thoughts of Hope and Comfort

A LOVELY LADY, PATRICIA MCNALLY, who wrote a beautiful book on angels and pregnancy called *Angelbumps*, recently told Dave and me that she could see a very strong presence around us. She said it looked like we have a guardian angel with us, keeping us safe and guiding us in the right direction. I got goose bumps when she said that to me. I literally felt a shiver down my spine. When I explained that we had lost a baby the year before, she did not look at all surprised. She said she could see a very strong presence of an angel around us and then she suggested that perhaps this presence was our baby. Perhaps our baby was lost in body but not in spirit. Perhaps our baby was still with us. I instantly felt like a weight had been taken off my shoulders. It is one of the most beautiful things anyone has ever said to me. I had been carrying a little bit of sadness with me since we had lost our baby and I honestly never thought it would leave me. But when Patricia suggested that our baby was still with us in spirit, I just felt that sadness wash away. Of course, I would always be sad that our baby did not make it into this world but the thought of our baby being here with us, even if it was in a way that we could not see or touch, was so comforting to me.

I personally don't know much about angels but I like to believe that what Patricia said to us is true. I like to think that if we have a guardian angel watching over us, it is our little baby. Before I had this thought, I often used to think back to that night when we actually lost the baby. It has always been very distressing for me to think back on that night. I am a very positive person and I think most things happen for a reason but I found it hard to come up with a reason for losing our baby. When awful things happen, I believe there is usually something good to come out of it. It might take a long time to learn whatever it was you were supposed to learn but there is usually something to learn. However, when we lost the baby I could not find anything good to focus on. I could not understand why this had happened and I just did not know what I was supposed to learn from it.

Now, when I look back on that difficult time, I think about all the ways in which that time challenged us, as individuals, as parents and as a couple. Now I can see all the things we learned from it.

I can see how it challenged my relationship with my husband but ultimately made us stronger. I can see how it challenged my relationships with family and friends but, somehow, we found a way to get through it, by talking about it. In some cases, like with one of my closest friends, Emma, it took three months before we sat down together properly and talked and cried about what had happened. The important thing is that we did sit down and talk and cry about it and, because of that, we got through it.

I realise now that it was this terrible event that made us so determined to have a better quality of life, which is why we moved house. We are so much happier where we live now and I sometimes wonder if we would have been so determined to move if it had not happened. Losing our baby also made us appreciate our son even more than we already did (which I did not think was even possible because we loved him so much already). It also made us so very, very excited when I became pregnant again. We cherished every minute of that pregnancy and are cherishing our lovely baby girl every day since she arrived.

Losing our baby gave us the drive to write this book together, in the hope that it will give some comfort to other mums and dads who have suffered the loss of their baby too. I could not have imagined writing a book so revealing and honest until this happened to us. It gave us the courage to be open and honest about our experience and not to be afraid to admit how we struggled. We share our experience in the hope it will make someone else going through it realise that there is light at the end of the tunnel.

The thought that our baby is a little angel who is still with us in spirit today gives me a sense of peace. It allows me to think that the baby's short lived time on this earth was not completely in vain. I feel happy when I think that my baby is still around in spirit. It comforts me to think this way, as it is a much better belief than the one I held previously. I used to think the baby was completely gone but now I think he or she is still around in a spiritual way. This thought gives me peace, hope and comfort and I don't think there's anything wrong with that.

If you have lost a baby and feel alone, sad or empty, just stop and think for a moment. Perhaps sometimes you can feel a presence around you. Perhaps your baby is still here in spirit too. This is not everyone's way of thinking and if someone had said this to me a few years ago I might have thought they were mad but now, just thinking that our baby's spirit is still with us, makes life easier for us, so we are happy to think this way. What's the harm if it gives us peace of mind and comfort? Perhaps thinking this way can bring you some comfort too. It's definitely a positive way to think of your baby's spirit.

Either way, please remember that there are lots of good things about life. There is something good in every day. You just need to recognise and appreciate the good things. It is so tempting to focus on the bad things, on the things that annoy or upset us. We have to learn to focus on the good instead. Sometimes life does seem harsh and unfair. That's why it is so important to look at the positive side of things. It is important to look forward to the future. It is imperative to have hopes and dreams. You must believe in yourself, so that you can achieve your hopes and dreams.

You can do whatever you want to, once you believe in yourself and keep your thoughts positive. Be good to yourself. Look after yourself. You are special and you should treat yourself the way you deserve to be treated. Read a good book; relax in a warm bath; take a long walk to clear your mind; go for a massage; give someone a hug; enjoy some retail therapy; have a romantic dinner with someone special. Do whatever it is that makes you feel calm and happy. Life is short, so enjoy it as much as you can, while you can. Don't dwell on the negative thoughts and sadness. Embrace your loss and remember your baby, but move on with your life. If you believe good things will happen to you, then they will.

As Eleanor Roosevelt once famously said: "The future belongs to those who believe in the beauty of their dreams." Dare to dream and dare to believe and you might just get what you wish for.

Epilogue

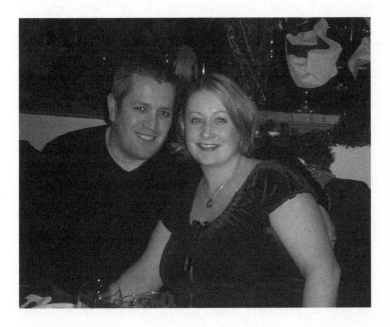

SIOBHÁN, DAVID, MITCHELL AND ROBYN live in Bettystown, on the coast in County Meath. Siobhán is currently working on her second book, *Nine Magical Months . . . and Then What?* This is a light-hearted story, based on the diary she kept during her first pregnancy. She writes part-time from home, so she can spend lots of time with the children.

David also works from home. He is a sales agent for an overseas property developer for Bulgaria. He travels abroad every month or so but mostly works from home, which enables him to spend a great deal of time with Siobhán and the children.

David and Siobhán are dedicated to their children and spend lots of time on the nearby beach, kicking football and chasing Mitchell and Robyn away from the waves. Despite their best efforts, they always come home soaking wet!

They are excitedly looking forward to the arrival of their third baby, who is due in July 2007.

Further Information

The Miscarriage Association of Ireland (Carmichael Centre, North Brunswick St., Dublin 7; phone: 01-8735702; website: www.miscarriage.ie

The Association is a charitable body set up by, and with the support of, women and men who themselves have been through miscarriages. They offer telephone support to bereaved parents, their families and friends and hold monthly support group meetings.

Your Local Hospital

Your local hospital may have a counselling service you can avail of; this service is usually free of charge and can be very helpful.

Your Local Health Centre

Health centres may have leaflets with information about miscarriage. You can get their numbers from the HSE (www.hse.ie).

Your Local GP

If you have feelings of despair, do not let them linger. Speak to your partner or family but if you cannot talk to them, or if it is not helping you to feel better, please contact your local GP. Do not be embarrassed; you are entitled to grieve and it takes a different amount of time for everyone, so if you feel you need help, please seek it out.

Counselling

If you do not wish to avail of the counselling services provided by your local hospital, you can seek out private counselling. Your GP can recommend someone suitable for you.

AWARE

You can contact AWARE, who offer advice for people suffering from depression. Visit their website at www.aware.ie